Nobody Is Listening: Stories of Inflammatory Breast Cancer

Patti Bradfield and Massimo Cristofanilli, MD

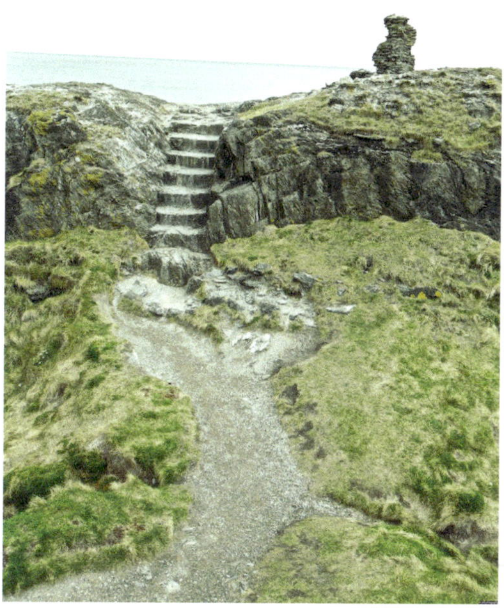

Bethesda Communications Group

Published by the Bethesda Communications Group
49 Wellesley Circle
Glen Echo, MD 20812
www.bcgpub.com

ISBN 13: 978-0-9761364-8-4
ISBN 10: 0-9761364-8-1

Photo credits
The cover photo and the photos illustrating the text were taken by Patti Bradfield, with the exception of the photo on page 84, which was provided by Kim Alexander.

Printed in the United States of America

All proceeds from the sale of this book go to support the IBC Foundation (www.eraseibc.com) and further their efforts to educate the public about IBC.

To Tina, Morgan, Angie, Lori and all the other IBC heroes

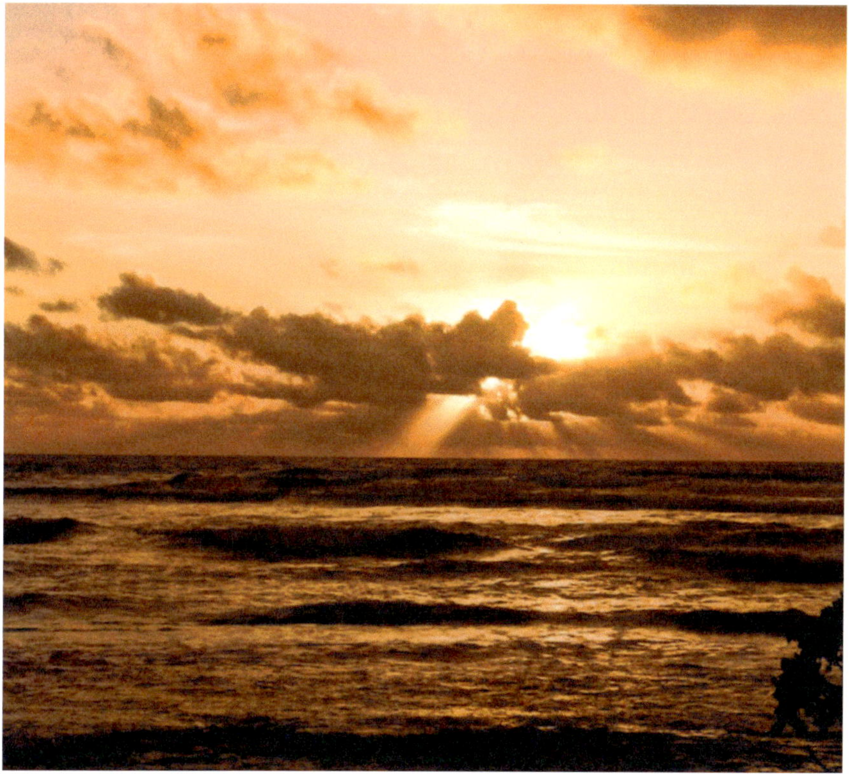

Contents

Preface

"We shall not fail or falter; we shall not weaken or tire... Give us the tools and we will finish the job.
Sir Winston Churchill

This book is not a work of fiction but a crude reality. Going through these pages you will find stories of ordinary women and their families who find themselves in a situation that they would have never imagined, facing an unknown killer disease for which nobody knows what to do.

It is the hope of each of these writers that their stories will inspire doctors, nurses, and the entire medical community to take more responsibility and understand that many times the most important aspect of their profession is the capacity to listen to their patients and always ask more questions and try to understand. This is particularly true when dealing with more rare and aggressive diseases such as inflammatory breast cancer (IBC).

It is also the hope from the compilers of this book that through the knowledge that is gained from reading these words, there will come an understanding of the cause and hopefully a cure for this devastating disease.

The idea for this work transpired from the lives of mostly women who never knew there was more than one type of breast cancer. Also, hopefully, you, the reader, will gain an inspiration from these pages of real life events. There is a breast cancer without a lump, and it is deadly.

Judge a man by his questions rather than by his answers.
Voltaire

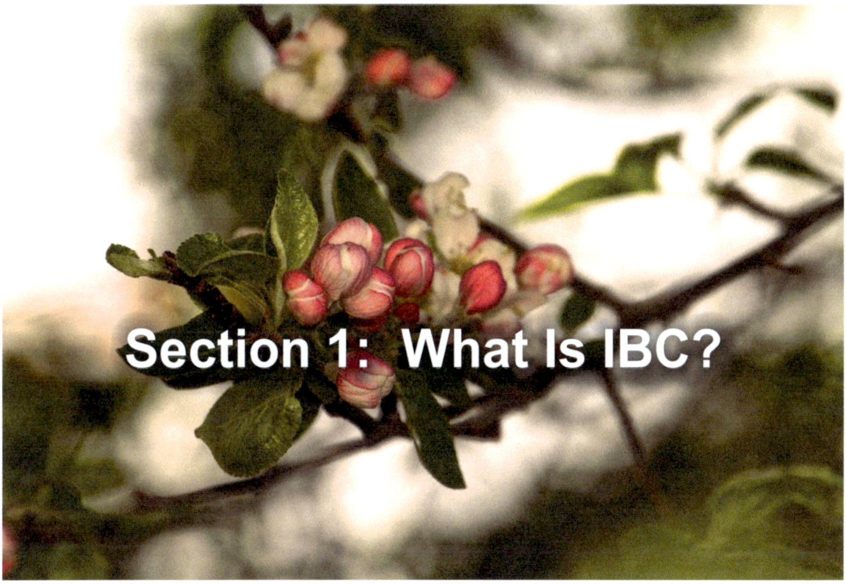
Section 1: What Is IBC?

IBC Facts

Inflammatory Breast Cancer (IBC) is the most aggressive type of breast cancer, in which the cancer cells block the lymph vessels in the skin of the breast. This type of breast cancer is called *inflammatory* because the breast often becomes swollen and red, or inflamed, sometimes overnight.

- IBC accounts for 1 to 5 percent (these numbers vary depending on their source) of all breast cancer cases in the United States. It tends to be diagnosed in younger women compared to non-IBC breast cancer.
- IBC lies in sheets (or nests), not the usual lump women are told to look for, thus rarely seen on routine mammograms.
- Inflammatory Breast Cancer occurs more frequently and at a younger age in African Americans than in Whites. The median age range of IBC patients is between 45 and 55 years old, but may be either younger or older.
- Like other types of breast cancer, IBC can occur in men.
- The 5-year median survival rate is approximately 40%, mainly due to delays in diagnosis, a physician's lack of expertise in treating IBC and its resistance to treatment with standard chemotherapy drugs.

IBC Signs and Symptoms

Because inflammatory breast cancer doesn't normally occur as a breast lump and has a peculiar growth pattern, its symptoms are not typical signs of cancer, and may appear to be an infection.

IBC symptoms may include one or more of the following:

- A breast that appears discolored; (red, purple, pink or bruised)
- A tender, firm and enlarged breast (sometimes overnight)
- A warm feeling in the breast (or may feel hot/warm to the touch)
- Persistent itching of the breast (not relieved with cream or salve)
- Shooting or stabbing pain
- Ridged or dimpled skin texture, similar to an orange peel
- Thickened areas of breast tissue
- Enlarged lymph nodes under the arm, above/below the collarbone
- Flattening or retraction of the nipple
- Swollen or crusted skin on the nipple
- Change in color of the skin around the nipple (areola)
- A hardened area in the breast similar to a pencil lead, not a lump

If one or more of these symptoms continue for more than a week, talk to a physician immediately and find an expert with experience in treating this particular type of breast cancer. Many women have to demand that their physicians "rule out" IBC, and therefore become their own best advocate, as more education is needed in the medical community regarding this form of breast cancer.

For more information, see the IBC Foundation website at www.eraseibc.com/ibc.html.

IBC, A Non-Clinical Definition

Cancer is like a sniper who can't shoot very well. Cancer can affect your body anywhere, usually in a non-lethal spot, but a somewhat debilitating spot nonetheless. You may recover most of your faculties, but now you know there's a sniper out there gunning for you—you don't know where it is or when it'll show up next or what part of you it'll get, but it's out there, ready to strike at any moment. So not only are you damaged physically, whether in a major or minor way, you're often haunted psychologically. And you know you can't be vigilant enough....

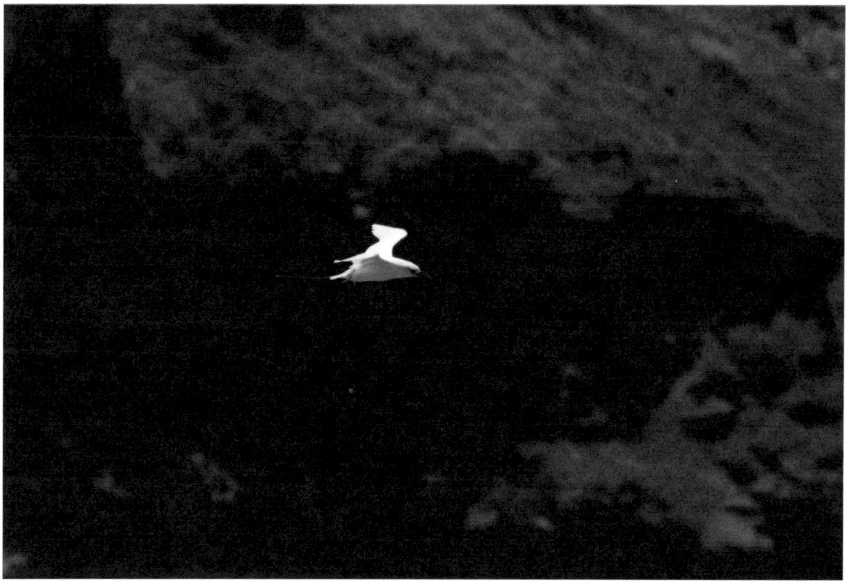

Some individuals are better than others in coping with the new reality after a diagnosis and treatment, and they usually will try to continue with their lives. This is only an apparent mask because you cannot ignore the sniper, and they just know the concern and the fear is always there, buried in the recesses of their minds and certainly causing underlying stress. Others, like me, want to talk a LOT about it and keep people's attention on it to make sure there's someone, anyone, trying to get rid of the sniper! It's the only way we can deal with the sniper and have any sense of control over the situation (whatever small control that may be). The sniper shot off my breasts and I've had shrapnel taken out, but I'm doing fine and I'm not letting the bastard take me out without a fight!!

Love & Peace, Chris (the Hoosier Hottie)

Ed. Note: Chris passed away on February 25, 2008. She was 54.

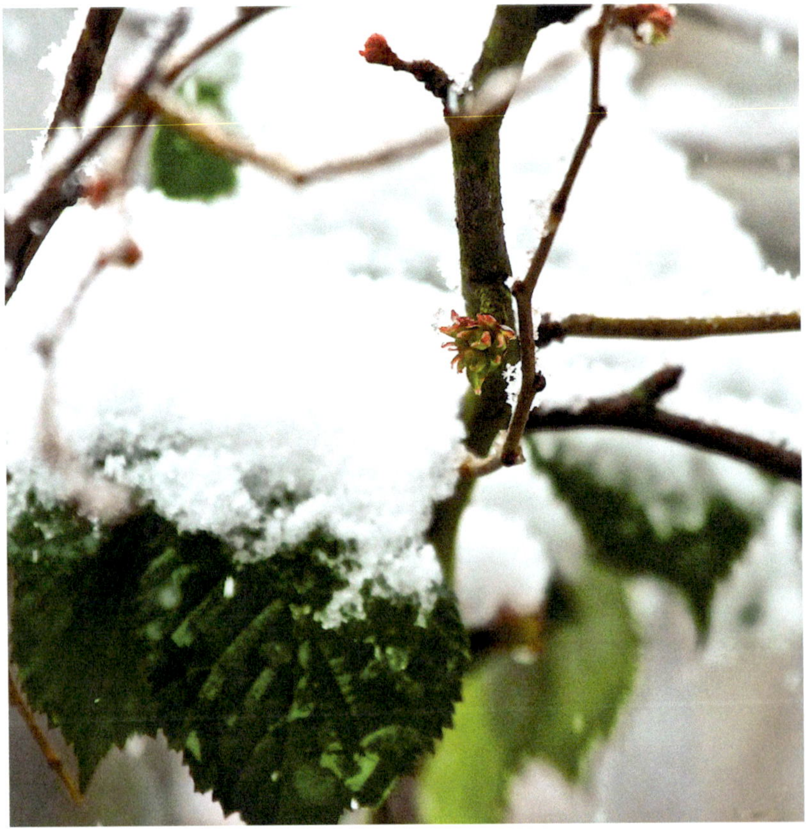

War of a Different Nature

Do not pray for easy lives. Pray to be stronger men.
John F. Kennedy

I didn't want to watch it. I knew I would cry again if I did. But of course I, like so many Americans, sat through another November 22 and watched our slain President Kennedy being moved off Air Force One, his wife in her pink blood-stained suit walking beside the flag draped casket. Walter Cronkite was taking his glasses off as the tears could not be hidden from the cameras while he told a nation, "President Kennedy has died." I wept that day and for the next 40 years every time I watched the replay and remembered.

On that fateful day in 1963, I was recuperating from a car accident, pregnant with my first child, and scared about what type of a country my child would be born into. I gave birth to a son, but he didn't go to war. Two years later I would have another child, this time a little girl, but she is now at war.

War against an enemy that has yet to be beaten. A criminal that no courts, no sniper's bullet, or army can seem to stop: CANCER!

Not just any cancer, but Inflammatory Breast Cancer (IBC), which has metastasized to her lymph nodes and liver. A cancer that some say is rare, but the numbers of women that have died from it doesn't seem to make it that rare.

In 1963 my world changed, as it did for so many people in America. We went from innocence to outrage. Well, it's 2003 and I am again outraged that a disease such as IBC is not talked about, written about, or fought in the open. It is just as much of a war as Vietnam was, or the war on terrorism is today. Just like those wars, IBC sneaks up on your body and by the time you know it's there, sometimes it's too late. You are already in the thick of the battle, and the weapons are not adequate to put it to a stop.

Ask yourself or anyone you know if they have heard of IBC. My guess will be they have not. We are told to look for a lump and to get mammograms.

We are not told there is another, sometimes undetectable, mass that there are signs of, if only we were told.

Like the march on Washington, DC, to stop the fighting in Vietnam, maybe there should be another march to decry an outrage that many physicians are not knowledgeable about or even aware of. We need to do some screaming to all young women that the old ways of looking at our bodies are as old as Vietnam and just as deadly.

Breast cancer, for the most part, hits older women. IBC seems to be more prevalent in young women in their child-bearing years, years when the doctors say you don't have to be too concerned about mammograms. IBC is hitting young girls in their late teens in some circumstances, and their mothers, like me, are so shocked that they never heard of this. Their emotions then go from shock to anger.

After I related my daughter's story to a pharmacist, she said, "Why haven't we been told about this so we could at least have the ability for early detection? This really makes me mad."

ANY DIFFERENCE in your breast, AT ANY AGE, should be looked at by a doctor who knows about this deadly disease. Don't let a doctor tell you that your 18-year-old daughter is too young for breast cancer, or it's probably a hormonal change or an infection. IBC moves in days, not months. It grows at such a rapid rate that some females have experienced an entire cup size difference in just one week. The American Cancer Society states that *"Inflammatory Breast Cancer lays in sheets and mammograms sometimes can't see any mass so the test comes back negative."*

If I have scared you by writing this, GOOD! I have accomplished something. Go on the Internet, to the library, or to a hospital and get the facts. Breast cancer is staged[1] from one to four. IBC is usually stage three or four and the prognosis is not good, but if you know that any change in the breast could possibly be cancer, early detection gives you more than a fighting chance.

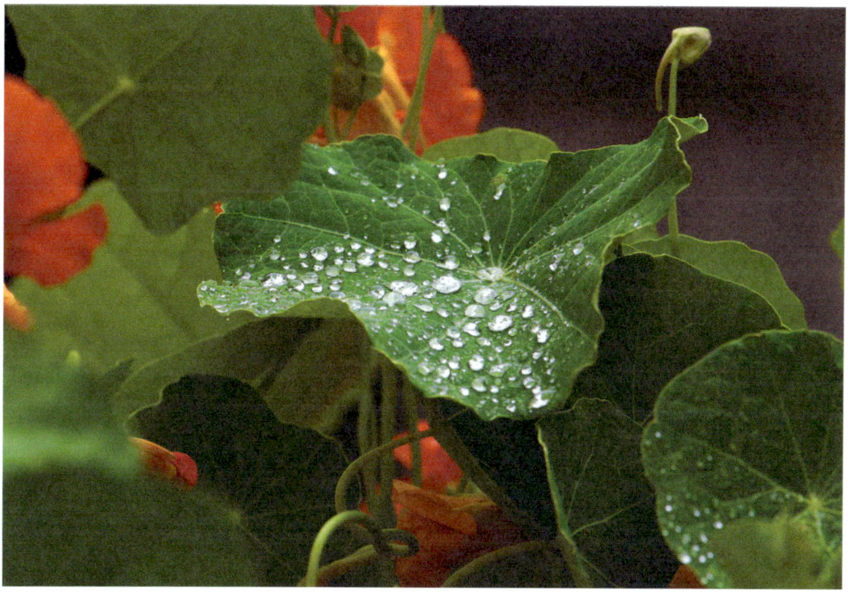

My terrified mind equates my daughter's fight to Vietnam or the war on terrorism. But this time around we have tools to fight with; we just need to know there is a war brewing and not be held back and kept in the dark as we have been in the past. We can't march on Washington with pink ribbons,

1 See *The Stages of Breast Cancer* in the next section.

but we can shout it out to anyone who will listen that IBC is amongst us and not be lulled into a delusional peace of mind that the young are safe from it.

My daughter was supposed to take care of me in my golden years. She might not see my golden years. AND THAT MAKES ME MAD!

Patti Bradfield, 2003

Ed. Note: Tina, Patti's daughter, tells her story in Section 2.

The Stages of Breast Cancer

Breast cancer can be divided into four numbered stages, which measure the size of the cancer and whether it's spread to the lymph nodes or another part of the body.

Stage 1—The cancer is smaller than, or equal to, 2cm and has not spread to the lymph nodes in the armpit.

Stage 2 is divided into two stages:

- Stage 2A—Either the lump is smaller than 2cm and has spread to lymph nodes in the armpit OR it's bigger than 2cm (but under 5cm) and hasn't spread to the lymph nodes OR the cancer can't be found in the breast but is in the lymph nodes in the armpit.
- Stage 2B—Either the lump is smaller than 5cm and has spread to the lymph nodes in the armpit OR it's bigger than 5cm but hasn't spread to the lymph nodes in the armpit.

Stage 3 is divided into three stages:

- Stage 3A—Either the cancer can't be found in the breast or the lump is under 5cm and the cancer is in the lymph nodes in the armpit, which are stuck together OR the lump is bigger than 5cm and has spread to the lymph nodes.
- Stage 3B—The cancer has spread to tissue near the breast and may be attached to surrounding skin or muscle. There are usually cancer cells in the lymph nodes in the armpit as well. Cancer that has spread to the skin of the breast may also be inflammatory breast cancer.
- Stage 3C—The cancer has spread to lymph nodes in the armpit, below the breastbone, near the neck or under the collarbone.

Stage 4—The cancer has spread to other parts of the body such as the bones, liver, or lungs. This is called metastatic breast cancer.

Grading

Grading refers to how the cancer cells look under the microscope compared with normal breast cells.

- Grade 1 (low-grade)—The cancer cells look similar to normal cells and grow very slowly.
- Grade 2 (intermediate-grade)—The cancer cells look more abnormal and are slightly faster growing.
- Grade 3 (high-grade)—The cancer cells look very different from normal cells and tend to grow quickly.

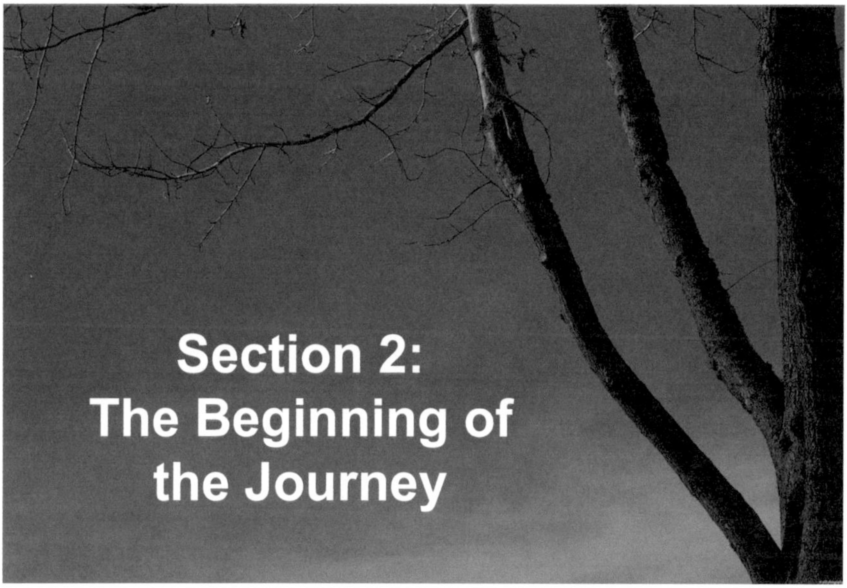
Section 2:
The Beginning of
the Journey

Moira's Story

Courage is being scared to death—but saddling up anyway.
John Wayne

Funny how a few little words can change your world. For me that happened just over two years ago, when a stranger said, "I think you have breast cancer—go out tonight and have a few drinks."

What he forgot to add was—you will lose your hair, self-confidence, control, normality, and you'll endure sleepless nights, pain, helplessness, despair, uncertainty, and anger, and on top of this have to deal with your family and friends' emotions whilst dealing with your own roller coaster ride and becoming an expert on cancer, treatments, and the drugs just around the corner that are going to prolong your life. And that the bottom line is that nothing will ever be the same again.

I don't think anyone truly appreciates what a cancer patient goes through, both physically and emotionally—I know I never did. Whenever I heard that someone's mother or grandfather had cancer—I passed on the necessary condolences and got on with my life and thought little more about it or how it affected them. Cancer wasn't part of my life plan.

Now that life of mine includes an amazing array of decisions and considerations. As a young woman with a terminal illness, I have other concerns—how will I financially support myself when I'm unable to work, should I and can I continue to work and if I can't, how will I survive? As a single person, who will look after me when I am no longer able to cope alone? As a patient, should I desperately try and get the latest trial drug or wait until I really need it? The endless list goes on and on.

I wish I'd never heard of Inflammatory Breast Cancer (IBC)—which officially found me on the 25th of January in 2005. But now that I have and understand its true significance, I'm keen to do as much as I can to ensure that it receives some attention—so that there are fewer people having to face the fears and uncertainty that I have had to.

My name is Moira—I am a 39 year old Australian lawyer currently living in the UK. I was 38 when diagnosed.

I will most likely die from IBC (unless that bus everyone keeps talking about to make me feel better gets me first) and this is my story.

In October of 2004 I was living in London—it's compulsory for every Australian to live for some time in the mother country. But after two years, the hectic pace of London had become too much for me and so I decided to move to Cheltenham, a pretty English town about two hours away.

Symptoms

About a month later—just as I'd moved into my beautiful apartment—I looked down one night and noticed I had an inverted nipple. I didn't think too much about it—just put it down to old age—but was curious as to how long it had been there without my noticing it.

It was only around Christmas when I started moving some furniture that I developed a pain in my breast—something I'd never experienced before. Around this time my breast started swelling and my skin looked like an orange peel. Little did I know then that I was exhibiting classic IBC symptoms. I still wasn't rushing to the doctor—how could I possibly have breast cancer? There was no family history and I was too young—plus there was no lump. It wasn't until I started putting my symptoms into a search engine on the Internet and I was directed to a breast cancer site that I thought I should seek medical attention. I visited a general practitioner. She didn't make too much of a fuss, just said it looked like mastitis, gave me antibiotics, and said she would refer me to the breast clinic "just in case."

I had an appointment with the breast clinic within two weeks, on the 25th of January in 2005, and that first appointment with my physician consultant blew me away. I had a physical examination, ultrasound, mammogram, followed by a biopsy—and it was at the end that my consultant told me those words that would change my world forever.

The diagnosis was officially confirmed the following Tuesday and the rest of the week was a blur—everything moved so quickly. I saw the oncologist the next day, had my pre-chemotherapy check up on the Thursday, and was booked in to start chemo on the Friday. As my partner and I were due to fly to Cuba that week, we agonized long and hard about whether to take the trip and delay treatment for two weeks. Though my consultant approved, my oncologist was keen to start chemo straight away. It was a confusing time—who do I listen to? Ultimately we cancelled our trip. I had concluded that if I delayed treatment even if only for two weeks and ultimately developed secondary breast cancer (which would mean it had metastasized to other parts of my body), could I live with myself and not kick myself for not starting treatment earlier?

Treatment

On the 9th of February in 2005 I started on a standard breast cancer chemotherapy drug combination—FEC[2]. My first infusion (of what was to be a total of six FEC) went fine—I was infused and out of the oncology ward by midday—but that was never to happen again and I have spent many, many hours hanging around the oncology ward. For those who aren't aware, having chemo isn't about just turning up every 3 weeks and getting some drugs—there's actually quite a lot that happens before that process. A usual day in oncology goes something like this: arrive around 9 am—wait—have blood taken—wait quite a bit—see oncologist to discuss side effects, blood results (you can only have chemotherapy if you have sufficient white and red blood cells). If the oncologist gives you the okay to have drugs—wait quite a long time whilst your prescription goes to the pharmacy and the chemo is made up and returned to oncology and a nurse is available to infuse you (this wait is usually several hours). Eventually get called in to be infused—the total infusion time depends on how long the chemo or other drugs are infused over. But I have to say I usually get to leave the oncology ward somewhere between 6 pm and 8 pm. It's a long day and not a particularly cheerful one, especially when I am usually the youngest person there. I hope people understand why I never look forward to my oncology days.

Anyway, after two rounds of FEC there appeared to be no change to the size of my swelling and my oncologist suggested a change to paclitaxel. I agreed, and although that meant another six cycles of this drug (on top of the original two FEC I'd already had—mentally a crushing blow), at least I saw almost immediate results on the paclitaxel—the swelling appeared to go down overnight.

I had decided to continue working throughout my

---

2 FEC is the name of a chemotherapy combination made up of the drugs Fluorouracil (5FU), Epirubicin, and Cyclophosphamide.

chemo—a decision which seemed to shock a few people. But I needed to continue to financially support myself and I had a supportive employer who would allow me to come into work when I felt like it. So my chemotherapy routine would be one week off work immediately following chemo, where I would take to my bed—then return to work for two weeks before the cycle started again. As a lawyer I had quite a mentally demanding job, and adjusting to the new crazy post-cancer diagnosis world was hard. But I found coming into work was the only bit of normal I had left from my previous life BC—before cancer. Thankfully I didn't suffer too much from chemo brain—a term used by those going through chemotherapy who have a tendency to forget things.

My partner resigned from his job and moved in with me—ironically I continued working to support us and he took care of the meals and house. It's a credit to him that I never had to delay a chemo due to having low blood counts. However at the end of six months of chemo I was feeling very weak—and missing my hair—I had not one hair on my body. I also thought that I looked quite ill or probably just as a cancer patient does. I remember being in the supermarket one day when I bent down to get something from the bottom shelf and I just had no strength in my legs and thought to myself, "I can't get up."

I had a short five-week break from the end of chemo to my surgery—a mastectomy—which is the standard treatment for IBC. It was during this time that I thought I'd better do some research about my cancer, as my friends had been encouraging me to do from the beginning. My oncologist had recently told me I had inflammatory breast cancer and one night at work I Googled it on the Internet.

The first thing I read was the overall survival statistics for IBC—a 40% chance of 5 year survival and almost no prospects of 10 year survival.

I felt like throwing up—I had no idea I had such a serious form of breast cancer. In fact, up until I started reading about breast cancer I had no idea there were different types—to me breast cancer was all about lumps and having a family history.

My mindset at the beginning was that I would have 12 months of treatment hell and then I would be "cured" and I'd just get on with my life—I didn't even think that this thing could actually kill me. Mentally it was a difficult time—it is isolating to be a young woman with breast cancer and to also have a rare form of the disease with such a grim outlook.

Thankfully I had a pre-surgery checkup with my consultant the following week and I had the opportunity for a long discussion with him—he was very good at giving me hope and saying it wasn't all doom and gloom. I felt slightly better. A couple of weeks later I had my pre-surgery mammogram—which was clear. Everyone thought this was great news and so did I—I recall going home that night and having my first proper sleep since IBC had entered my life.

Unfortunately it didn't last long—my post-surgery pathology showed microscopic traces of cancer in the breast, and I had 4 to 16 lymph nodes infected. I was gutted, as my consultant was away and the news was delivered by the breast care nurse who kind of indicated that it was bad and I was going to die. It took a long time mentally to get over my pathology results.

It was around this time that I discovered the IBC support group, which I immediately joined. I was welcomed by a supportive and loving group of men and women who more importantly, by sharing their stories, gave me hope—something I hadn't had in a long time.

After a four-week break following my mastectomy, I returned to work—I had decided at the time to have an immediate reconstruction in my IBC breast and a reduction in my left good breast—quite major surgery. Around this time Herceptin was all abuzz in the UK media for treatment of early stage breast cancer, though not licensed nor funded through the public health system in the UK. My partner and I agreed to privately fund Herceptin, costing us around £30,000, which was a lot of money, but we figured the increased prospects of my survival statistics were worth it.

Given that Herceptin was in the news constantly, the government was under a great deal of pressure to make this drug available—the end result being that my local hospital agreed to fund the drug on my behalf.

Three months after my surgery, I started radiotherapy—a total of 15 treatments over five weeks, which I completed in early December. I was due to start my three weekly Herceptin infusions in January of 2006 and was excited for even this small break from treatment, though by this stage I had started the dreaded tamoxifen—a daily tablet drug which tries to suppress estrogen production in my body, as my cancer was estrogen receptor positive. This is not a pleasant drug, though my side effects were relatively mild—some hot flushes and night sweats, though it was the mood swings which I found difficult to cope with. It was not helpful that a week before Christmas of 2005, my partner of three years unexpectedly ended our relationship—this was a difficult time as I now had to face being a young woman with a mastectomy entering the dating world again—a daunting prospect on top everything else I'd been dealing with.

And it happened at a time when I was just enjoying getting over the initial treatment and being NED—No Evidence of Disease—which is the hope of every cancer patient. Contrary to popular belief, you are never *cured* of cancer as such—the most you can hope for is that there is no evidence of the disease—and the longer you remain NED, the more your survival statistics improve.

I started Herceptin in January of 2006 and was due to have 12 months—I viewed my day in oncology every three weeks to receive treatment as an inconvenience as I sought to try to get on with my life being NED. Everything seemed to be going along fine until I developed an abscess in my reconstructed implant in May of 2006. I hadn't been feeling well for a while, but put it down to my stressful job and having the flu on top of an ear infection.

Unfortunately the abscess erupted and I was hospitalized for two weeks—this was the start of three months in and out of the hospital as my consultant sought to control the infection and save my implant. The day before my initial admission I had developed a throbbing pain just under my left rib cage. It felt slightly better after the abscess was drained—but I casually mentioned it to one of the ward doctors. A bone scan was ordered but I was told it was just precautionary. I didn't think too much about it.

At this stage I was attending the hospital every second day to have my abscess wound dressed and on the 27th of July in 2006 I turned up for my appointment as normal. The doctor came to see me, dressed the wound, and told me that they had my bone scan results. She then placed her hand on my knee and I knew then that the news was not going to be good. I was told that my cancer had spread to my bones. I was completely floored—I just wasn't prepared for that news. I was told my treatment plan was to continue on with Herceptin, with the addition of another drug—a bisphosphonate pamidronate—to prevent calcium leaking from my bones. I was whisked down for more blood tests—I remember getting in straight away and ahead of a lot of people waiting—but I guess when you get bad news, you deserve a bit of special treatment. I had my blood test and walked home sobbing my eyes out and I really didn't care who saw me.

I had read enough about breast cancer to know that any cancer that had spread or metastasized, also known as secondaries, was not good and that ultimately I would die from this disease. That's a very hard piece of news to hear when you are 38 years of age.

It took some time to adjust to my bone cancer spread—but I continued working and furiously researching (and had convinced myself I could survive a decade even with bone spread), when on the 27th of September I was told the news that every cancer patient dreads—further scans revealed that the cancer had spread to my liver.

Now I was really freaking out—I knew that would mean more chemotherapy—something I'd hoped I'd never have to go through again—and that my situation was becoming more serious. My oncologist talked about this being a "setback," not "death," and we discussed the many treatment options that were still available to me. That's what I like about my oncologist—he never gives up hope for me. I eventually decided to start on Xeloda, an oral non-balding chemo—as I had planned a trip home to Australia at Christmas and I didn't want to return home bald.

I have now completed cycle four and I am currently awaiting further scan results to see if the chemotherapy is working. I'm not sure how I will cope if it isn't, but I guess I'll have to. Encouragingly my skin metastases (which I developed shortly after my bone diagnosis) seem to be healing. Since the diagnosis of my metastases, I have continued to work full time—just having the day off to attend treatment in oncology every three weeks. Thankfully I am handling the Xeloda chemo quite well and I'm able to return to work the following day, with manageable side effects of mild nausea, fatigue, and blisters on my hands and feet. I do tend to sleep a fair amount on the weekends though.

People often comment about how “brave” I’ve been or that I seem to be handling everything in a manner that they never could. I don’t think so—of course there are days when I have uncontrollable sobbing fits about everything. But generally I find it’s just so surreal, it’s like its happening to someone else. I just try to get on with the normal in my life—going to work, being social, and having as much fun as I possibly can. The thing I find about cancer is that you get the bad news in increments, so that your mind has time to process the news and adjust to the new normal.

So that’s where I am at—39 years of age facing a terminal illness. Nine years ago a good friend of mine died from melanoma. I recall commenting at the time about how in some ways knowing you were going to die might be a good thing, as it gives you the opportunity to say goodbye and do those things you always wanted to do before you go. Now that I’m facing it myself I can assure people that my view has most definitely changed—there isn’t one second of one day since the 25th of January in 2005 that I haven’t thought about cancer. The uncertainty that cancer brings—in terms of treatment, choices, decisions, future—are some of the hardest things to deal with.

Epiphany

I had an epiphany the other day—I decided that I was approaching my early demise in the wrong way. I had been despairing of the brutal unfairness of it all—especially getting it so young and at a time when I feel the most confident in myself. Some days those thoughts were so completely overwhelming that I had no idea how to deal with them without uncontrollable sobbing and getting so angry. But I have decided to think about it another way: Have I only gained this confidence and self-appreciation of the person I am and want to be because of my cancer experiences? If so, then I am in a better position than someone who doesn't have that introspection and dies miserable.

Who knows if that is the case, but those thoughts work for me for today.

Ed. Note: Moira passed away on May 8, 2007. She was 39.

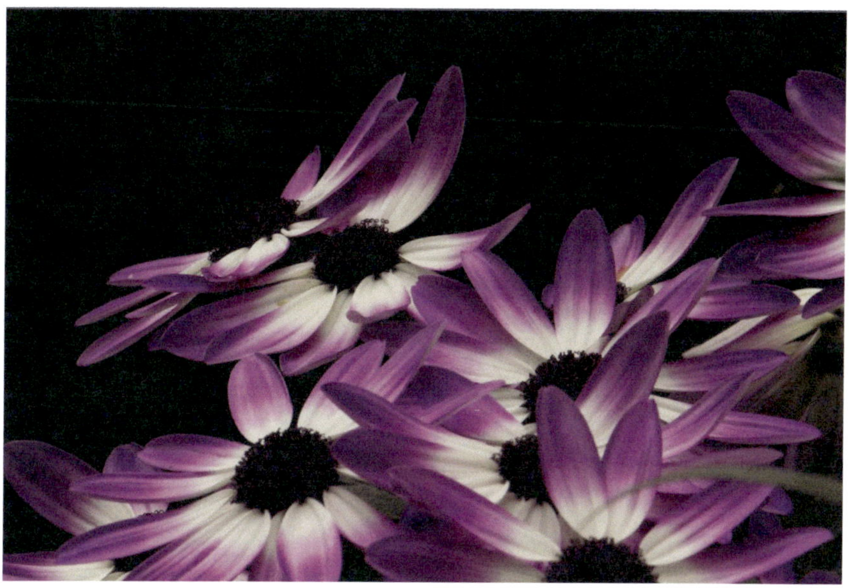

Marijanne's Story

Symptoms

This is the concise summary of my story. During the summer of 2005, my right breast suddenly looked larger and had a swollen look. I checked for lumps and stared at it for minutes at a time. It looked strange but felt fine. A few weeks later, in early fall, the right breast was very itchy and I could not get my right arm to be comfortable. I felt discomfort wearing my seat belt. I was constantly trying to readjust it.

Diagnosis

I remember on October 13, 2005, I went in for my yearly mammogram as soon as insurance would cover it. I felt something was wrong—my breast felt very hard, was turning red, and still had the swollen, itchy, uncomfortable feeling. The mammogram tech said everything looked good and I felt a major relief. The tech had asked for a physician to look at me because my breast looked strange. The doctor came in, examined my breast and quickly said, "You should get to a breast surgeon, do not pass go, do not collect $200. Get somewhere quickly." I saw a surgeon the next day, and he told me to go home and get prepared for a diagnoses of cancer. How in the heck do you do that? He called the following Friday night around 7:00 pm and he was talking very fast, telling me I had breast cancer. He kept repeating the word "inflammatory." I was confused. What does inflammation have to do with breast cancer?. I went to the net, typed in a Google search, three words that forever changed my life. The three words I chose were Breast Cancer Inflammatory. I stayed up that night getting information, sitting in disbelief!

Things started happening fast after that: I got a second

opinion and decided to go with the Medical College of Virginia and with a physician who had a great reputation. I had the port[3] installed in late October by a surgeon whom I love.

A little about me, I was 49 when I was diagnosed—the mother of two girls 11 and 13 years old, married, and with a full-time job. I carry the benefits. I needed to get treatment close to home. Other than having kids late in life and starting my period early (at age 12), I had no other "risk" factors. I exercised daily and ate right.

Treatment

My chemotherapy started on November 3, 2005. I was started on Docetaxel once every three weeks. When me and my bald self went in for a checkup, they thought the breast looked a little smaller but they did not get the results they were hoping for, so I got another dose of Docetaxel. I went back in three weeks and the beast actually looked like it was growing, looking more red and swollen. I was told that was not a good sign. I started another chemotherapy, AC,[4] every other week.

After the first treatment, things looked pretty good and after the second one my breast looked somewhat "normal." We were celebrating. The chemotherapy treatments were

---

3 A port, or portacath, is a device that is installed under the skin in the upper chest. It consists of a reservoir (the portal) and a tube (the catheter). The portal is implanted under the skin in the upper chest for patients who need frequent or continuous administration of chemotherapy drugs. The drugs are delivered into large central vein where they are diluted by blood stream and delivered efficiently to the entire body.

4 AC is named after the initials of the chemotherapy drugs used. These are doxorubicin, which was originally known as Adriamycin®, and cyclophosphamide.

completed in February of 2006. The MRI showed no cancer. I went to surgery and I had a modified mastectomy on March 17. I requested a double mastectomy but I was told there was less than a 5% chance the cancer would go to the other breast. Pathology showed residual cancer in five nodes (only five were taken), cancer in the breast tissue, and cancer in the skin of the breast. I started twice a day radiotherapy in April. I had a checkup around the middle of June and things looked good. I flew to Atlanta for a business trip right after the checkup. I was sitting in the airport on my way home and felt an enlarged node above my collar bone. I called my physician the following Monday, and I went in to have it checked out. It came back positive for IBC, and the scans showed that the disease was present in two nodes above the right collar bone and in one more node under my left arm. I started on Xeloda the first of July and shortly thereafter the nodes appeared to be shrinking. I woke up in early September to find that the left breast was looking swollen and immediately I called my physician. IBC was now present in left breast, plus the nodes appeared to be getting larger. I started a new chemotherapy, Gemzar/Cisplatum, in early September. During this time I decided to get a third opinion about the management of my disease, and I went to the Dana-Farber Cancer Institute. They confirmed that I was receiving an appropriate treatment. By late November the left breast was still looking red and swollen and it was starting to itch. The scans showed the same three nodes and a spot on my liver. Once again I switched the chemotherapy cocktail, this time to Taxol/Avastin, taken weekly for 12 weeks straight. I completed my fifth treatment last Thursday and I am just starting to get some energy and will be heading in for my sixth treatment this week (if my counts hold up). I am told this is not a cure but may prolong my life. Currently it appears to be working. I'll go off this combo by the end of February and I will continue to have checkups to see where IBC will appear next. I'm hoping it won't be back for months—I could use a break from all this chemotherapy. Plus, it would be nice to have a little hair for a while.

Ed. Note: No followup information is available for Marijanne.

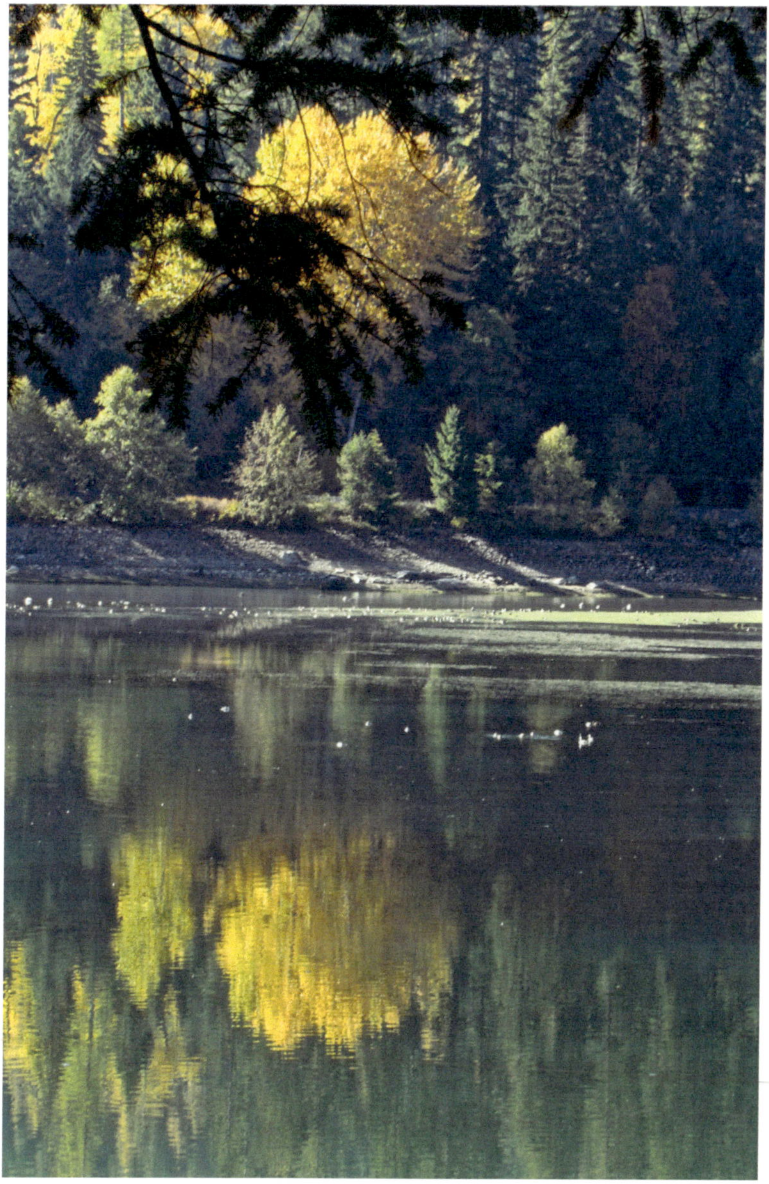

ɔan's Story

My name is Joan. I am a breast cancer survivor. I feel especially fortunate because the type of breast cancer I had was inflammatory breast cancer, a very rare and dangerous type of breast cancer.

Symptoms

It was February or March of 1995, at age 54, when I noticed in the bathroom mirror my right breast had a reddened area, circular in shape and about the size of a small orange on the medial side of the nipple area. It was not hot to the touch or painful. I was working as a hospital RN at the time on the gynecology surgery unit.

Initial Treatment

That day at work, I mentioned the problem to the nurse making rounds for my OB/GYN doctor. She called the office and made an appointment for me to see one of the associates that afternoon. That physician took one look and put me on antibiotics. I was told to return in one week if there wasn't any improvement. A week later there was absolutely no improvement so I went back and was able to see my regular doctor. He took one look and immediately said I needed to see a surgeon. This was all without any explanation as to why I should see a surgeon.

Followup Testing

I called a surgeon I had known for a number of years and made an appointment for the next day. When he saw my breast, he said he suspected breast cancer and scheduled me for an incisional biopsy a few days later. The biopsy was done and all the pathology results were negative. He admitted he was baffled by this outcome because it was not what he expected. He spent the next few weeks talking with any doctor who would listen about my condition and looking for suggestions as to what approach to take. One other surgeon suggested I stop taking Premarin. I had been taking only the lowest dose available for about eight months prior to the inflamed breast. I stopped taking the Premarin and the redness seemed to fade. Then my surgeon decided to get married and went on a two-week honeymoon.

Meanwhile, I was still waiting. By then it was July and I made a trip to my see my grandson be christened. While driving home, I felt discomfort in my armpit on the right side and there had developed a golf ball sized soft lump on the lateral side of the nipple area inside the breast.

Diagnosis

As soon as I got home, I made another appointment with the surgeon. He felt the lump and proceeded to do a "punch" biopsy of the area. The results from that biopsy took several days and also proved to be negative for any cancer cells. Again, we were waiting, with little to no direction as to what to do next. The breast continued to become more swollen and uncomfortable.

It was decided to do a much larger wedge biopsy from a different area of the breast. This incision was nearly 3 inches long, whereas the first was much smaller. Days went by and I finally heard from the surgeon. The pathologist had reported numerous slides had been made from the specimen and there were no cancer cells. My surgeon wasn't going to give up (thank God) and told the pathologist to keep making slides until the whole specimen had been used if that was what it took. Finally on the fiftieth and fifty-first slides there were positive cells for inflammatory breast cancer. The pathologist was amazed that it took that many slides and then he only found a few cells. But at least the diagnosis could finally be made and I could be referred to an oncologist.

I had my first meeting with the oncologist almost six months after the first signs of a problem. He spent a lot of time going over the plans for treatment with me. My husband convinced me we should get a second opinion. I was set up for a consultation at the MD Anderson Hospital at the Texas Medical Center in Houston, TX. I live about 30 miles from that medical center. The doctors there concurred that the diagnosis was correct and the treatment plan was appropriate. My local oncologist was actually in the MD Anderson system as an associate physician. So I opted to have my treatment close to home. I personally knew the nurses in his office, and being an employee of the hospital I would be using was comfortable for me.

Treatment

We started treatment in September of 1995. I had three months of chemotherapy with FAC (5-FU, Adriamycin, Cyclophosphamide). I lost my hair about two weeks after the first chemo treatment. My grown daughter, Laurie, very much a believer in home remedies using herbs and supplements, had purchased the book *Beating Cancer with Nutrition* by Patrick Quillin, 1994 edition. (The book has been revised since.)

Using this book as a guide, she made a list of supplements which I started taking several times a day when I started the chemotherapy. I believe doing so helped improve my energy level and state of general health. I continued to work at the hospital most of the time during my treatment.

The first of December I had a modified radical mastectomy.

A few days after my surgery, I developed an infection at the drain sites and was rushed to the hospital with sepsis. I was on IV antibiotics for five days before they were able to isolate the bacteria. It was very rare and had a name way too long to remember. I was discharged on home antibiotic therapy. Then my Groshong catheter became unusable. The day after Christmas I was back in the hospital to have the catheter removed and a portacath implanted.

Three more months of chemotherapy followed, complete with sore mouth and lack of appetite. I didn't suffer from nausea, but I just didn't feel like eating. After completing the chemo, I was scheduled for 26 treatments of radiation therapy, five days a week. Because I had been treated with Adriamycin, I suffered from burns at the breast area that were very painful. The area also wept and would stick to clothing, etc. I found Advanced First Aid™ 2nd Skin Moist Burn Pads applied to the open areas a life saver. I used these for several weeks while the area healed.

Finally in May 1996, I thought I was through with treatment. My oncologist had other plans. He wanted to give me four treatments of Taxol chemotherapy for good measure. I took the first treatment, and 48 hours later my left leg wouldn't work right, I felt like I was going to fall all the time and I hurt in every joint and bone in my body. I refused to take any more of that particular drug.

Treatment for the other breast

My hair grew back and my follow-up scans and lab work were all looking good. Home free, or so I thought. Near the end of May, 1997, I discovered in the mirror again, my left breast was inflamed and red just like a "mirror" image of the right breast two years prior. What a kick in the stomach. Probably the most devastating day of my life. I called my oncologists office and went to see him. It was decided not to bother with chemotherapy, but for me to go immediately into surgery for another modified radical mastectomy. In June, I had that surgery. Then I was scheduled for eight treatments of Taxotere and Navelbine chemotherapy.

The side effects of these drugs affected me greatly. I developed extreme pain in my back and joints within 24 hours of a treatment. I had to take Vicodin and sleeping pills to survive. I also had neuropathy in my feet and hands. The odd sensations are still present in my feet nine years later. Because of the toxicity of these drugs, I had to take huge amounts of Decadron prior to each treatment. That drug caused my eyes to develop cataracts to the point where I had to have lens implants done in 1998. I suffered from what I called "nerve shocks." I would be just sitting on the couch and have these shocks of pain shoot up through my legs. After I stopped the chemo, these took several weeks to disappear. I talked my oncologist into canceling the last chemo treatment. I was just so miserable.

My body has an innate ability to produce large amounts of scar tissue. Every place where I have had an incision is tight with scar tissue and I have spasms in my chest wall. The last portacath was surrounded with scar tissue and became swollen and painful. I couldn't wait to get it removed. The surgeon said he had a difficult time closing the incision because the scar tissue was so aggressive. For the second time, I had 26 radiation therapy treatments, this time without the skin burns. What a relief.

Now I am 11 years from diagnosis of the first breast and 9 years from diagnosis of the second breast, and after much research about IBC, I realize I am lucky to be writing my story. Six months for that first diagnosis could have been my death sentence. I had never heard of IBC in all my years of nursing. Even the oncologist's office nurse told me she went home and looked in her books to find out what IBC was. She had not treated a single patient with that diagnosis. I met a young lady in her 30's who was a patient of my oncologist and who was diagnosed with IBC the same year I was. She was pregnant at the time of her diagnosis. They did treatment and the baby was fine. However, she developed skin metastases and she was on chemotherapy for the next 7 years. She lost her battle with the demon when she was only 38 years old. It was so sad. She left a husband and two beautiful boys.

I am so blessed to be here on earth, but it's been a battle. I have suffered with clinical depression, weight gain, bilateral lymphedema, and the side effects of Tamoxifen and Fareston. But at least I am here to complain about the swollen arms, etc.

Lymphedema is my other "soap box" topic. In this country of highly skilled medical professionals, there is a huge lack of knowledge about this topic.

We have limited sources for treatment and support.

I know that the treatment for IBC has much improved since I went through my therapy and the success rate is probably higher. I hope this is true.

At the time of this writing, my tumor markers are normal with no signs of metastases.

Ed. Note: No followup information is available for Joan.

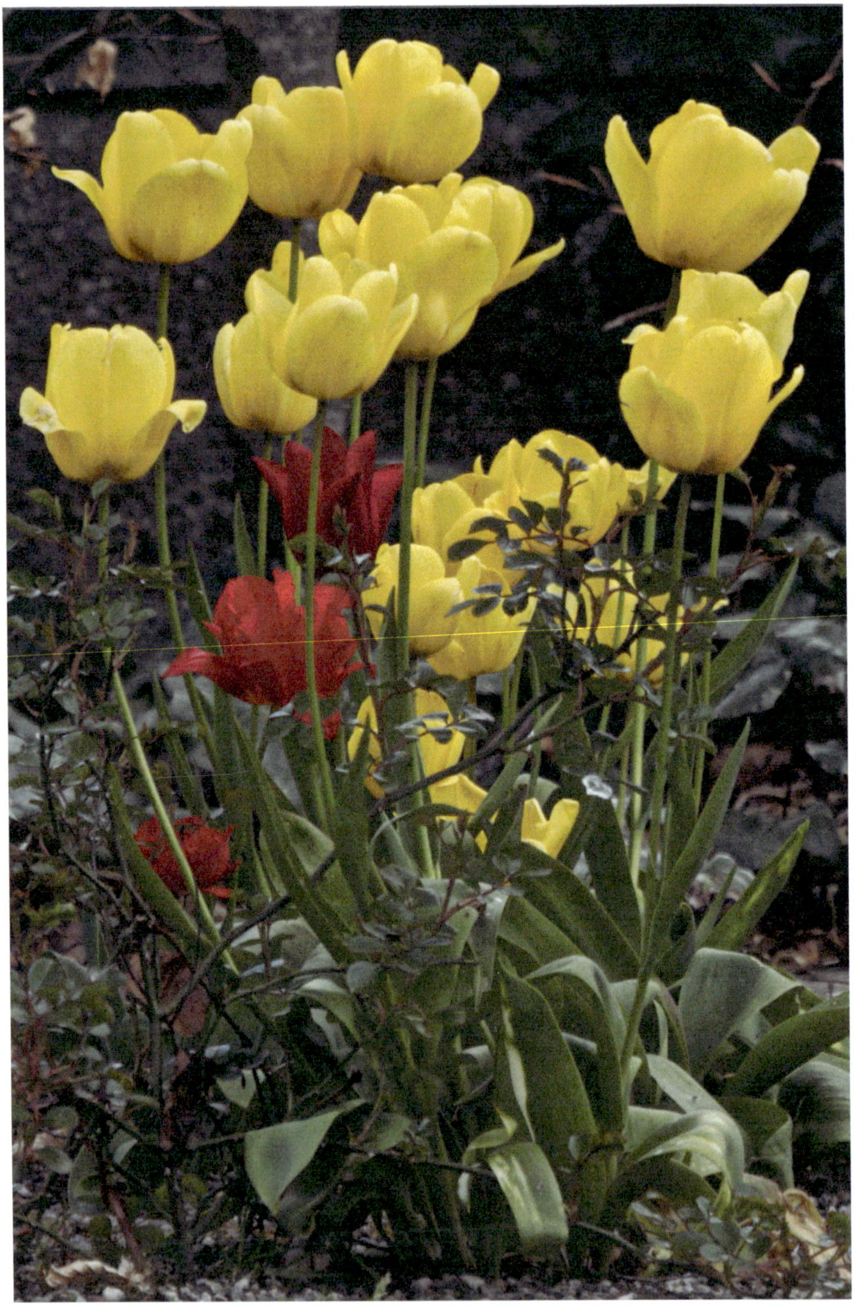

Deby's Story

Courage is resistance to fear, mastery of fear
—not absence of fear.
Mark Twain

When did IBC take over my life? I am a 48-year-old female with a strong family history of breast cancer on the paternal side of my family. I don't drink or do drugs of any kind. I am active with our boys and walk regularly 30 minutes a day. I think we eat pretty nutritionally, but I have been overweight on and off most of my life.

My sister and I have always been told that we are at no greater risk of breast cancer than any other female because breast cancer was on the paternal side of our family. We have both fought to get mammograms earlier than the recommended starting age, but the insurance companies or doctors would not do mammograms any earlier.

My fight with IBC started late in March of 2006. The first symptom I had was just a pain in my left breast that wouldn't go away and what I though was enlarged pores and now know to be peau d'orange. I would take over the counter pain medications like ibuprofen and Tylenol as advised by my family doctor. The pain persisted. So, I called to get an appointment with my doctor, who's first available appointment was three weeks out, so I saw another physician in the same clinic. The first appointment I could get was in April since I didn't have a lump or a serious problem.

The physician did a breast exam, finding no problem: no lump, no swollen lymph nodes, nothing visually unusual with my breast. She suggested I take birth control pills to help with the pain, which was probably from hormone changes. I asked if this could be anything else and she stated "No" and told me not to worry since breast cancer never had pain associated with it and I had no other signs of breast cancer. I asked that we do another mammogram because I had such a strong family history of breast cancer. Since my previous mammogram was just six months earlier, we had to have that approved by my primary physician and Kaiser. It took almost two months of phone calls before I could get the approval for another mammogram. (The pain and the peau d'orange still had not gone away.)

Finally, on June 6, 2006, I went for the mammogram and was told I'd get a letter in the mail. When after two weeks the letter hadn't come, I started calling to find out the results of my test. I was told that my films had been lost and no one had read them. The breast clinic had also lost my previous films and didn't have anything to compare the new films to, so nothing had been done!

I finally got a phone call stating that they wanted to do another mammogram on July 2. I went to have the mammogram and the technician said to me; "What is that?" referring to the peau d'orange and some redness. She did the mammogram and told me to dress and wait in the waiting room. Then I was told they wanted to do an ultra sound, which they did.

Then the physician who read the ultra sound came in and told me that I had breast cancer. There was no compassion, no buffer, no comfort…just: "You have cancer!" I was stunned! I didn't know what to ask, what to do, where to go. The physician said that because of what they saw on the mammogram and the ultrasound, they wanted to do a needle biopsy as soon as possible.

I left to drive home, stunned as I was, to break the news to the love of my life. I never felt so alone in my life!

I had the needle biopsy and met with a surgeon, who explained the treatments for breast cancer. He was ready to set up a surgical appointment, but then noticed the peau d'orange. He did another biopsy for "something suspicious." Once again I was told to go home and wait for another phone call. The surgeon finally called us and told my husband that the skin biopsy showed that I had a "high risk breast cancer" called inflammatory breast cancer (IBC) and that the treatment for that was different and that they didn't know if they would ever do surgery. He told us that I had little hope of surviving IBC long term. Our next step would be to meet with an oncologist, for which we also had to wait for a phone call…it just seemed that no one was taking this seriously…at every turn we had to WAIT for a phone call… if the IBC didn't kill me, the continuous wait for a phone call would.

I got on the computer and did some research. Most of the information gave me little hope for survival more than two or three years, stating that 50 percent of IBC cases don't make it past five years. I started imagining all the things I wouldn't see….I have a wonderful husband and two sons ages 12 and 19…graduations, marriages, grand babies, lives fulfilled. I was destroying myself in a bucket of frustrations and tears. I needed to get myself together and start helping myself.

It was now the middle of July, almost 4 months since I was first seen about my breast pain and we were still waiting to see the oncologist. I was afraid that the longer we waited, the more the cancer would spread.

I was getting more and more frustrated with the "care" I was not getting from Kaiser. So I decided to take things into my own hands. I called every hospital in the Portland, Oregon, area and asked which hospital has the best breast cancer treatment center. Most of those hospitals directed me to Oregon Health Sciences University (OHSU). So I called the OHSU breast care clinic and spoke with an oncology nurse who is an angel on earth. She asked me questions, showed real concern, and got me an appointment the next day with three of their best breast cancer physicians, including an oncologist. I went to Kaiser and got all the films, tests results, and chart notes. I also called my surgeon to ask for a referral to OHSU for a second option and was turned down.

I went to OHSU anyway and paid for it myself. At first the physicians at OHSU thought I didn't have IBC, but the skin biopsy results and their examination showed that I did have IBC, though it seemed to be a very slight case. The doctor at OHSU told me exactly what to tell the oncologist at Kaiser to do. He thought that I should do the TAC regimen every three weeks for six treatments, to be followed up with surgery and radiation. He told me tell Kaiser I needed an immediate Muga test, a bone scan, and a CT scan, and he told me that there was hope that I could survive this by keeping strong and active throughout my chemo treatments. The nurses, physicians, and oncologist at OHSU gave me more information and more hope than I ever had from any interaction at Kaiser. My husband and I left that hospital with renewed hope and a game plan that we knew was going to save my life. I'm sure you could have seen a happy skip in our walk.

Immediately after that visit I called the Kaiser oncology department head and insisted that I set up a chemo start date. I was in control now! I didn't want to meet with the oncologist just to end up waiting for a week or two in order to get this all set up. The department head stated that was not how they did things, that the normal procedure was to meet with the oncologist, make a treatment plan, and then schedule the first chemo treatment. I told her I didn't have normal breast cancer—I have IBC and I've already waited too long! She made a chemo appointment for July 31. I was happy just to be getting something going.

My oncology appointment started out with a surprise visit to the cancer counselor. I was upset at the department head for not telling us about it first. After an hour with the cancer counselor we were finally ushered to see the oncologist, who told us that OHSU had forwarded the recommended treatment plan to him. He thought it would be safer to do Adriamycin and Cyclophosphamide every two weeks for six treatments and then Taxotere every two weeks for six treatments to be followed up by surgery and radiation. We had to insist that we wanted to do the TAC as suggested by OHSU and all the other tests that OHSU said I should be having for staging and to figure out exactly what we were fighting. (All the scans came back normal.) The oncologist finally agreed only IF my tests for the Her2 came back before my July 31 chemo treatment. Luckily the test results came back before chemo and we started the TAC treatments every three weeks for six treatments. The tests showed that I was a triple negative: hr-/pr-/her2u—only confirming that the TAC regimen was the right treatment. We needed to be aggressive like the disease. I was strong, determined, and ready to go!

In August, I was tested for a possible gene mutation, which was confirmed in October when the results came back.

Every time I'd have a chemo treatment, we'd meet with the oncologist who would confirm that the lymph nodes and lump were getting smaller to the point where they could no longer be felt—the TAC was working ! Sure I'd lost my hair, lost some weight, and lost my appetite, I couldn't go out into the sun, and I slept a lot, but I was fighting this beast and was happy to be doing it, no matter what the side effects—I'm a strong, bald, and beautiful woman, ready to win this fight.

The surgery that followed was a breeze compared to chemo, and my new surgeon was wonderful! He was positive that the surgery would be successful and felt that since I had such a good response to chemo, I should have no problem with recovery from surgery. I was positive, strong, and ready to get this surgery done! I had a double mastectomy because of the gene mutation. The lab reports showed I had no cancer in either breast and the sentinel node biopsy on my right side came back clear also. Two lymph nodes, however, on my left (IBC) side came back positive for cancer. I started my second round of chemo on January 7, 2007, doing Taxol and Gemzar every two weeks for four treatments. This was part of our original treatment plan all along (as suggested by me). Once the two nodes showed up with cancer, we knew the second round of chemo was the right thing to do. I was scheduled to start radiation treatment in early March after I finished my last chemo treatment.

Once I took control of my cancer treatment by getting that second option, I stopped letting myself be the victim. I changed my mindset to think myself well, be positive, and fight for myself. I've also realized that nothing in the world is more valuable than every moment of my life, and I'm not going to give anyone else the power to take that away from me without a fight.

Ed. Note: Deby continues to thrive.

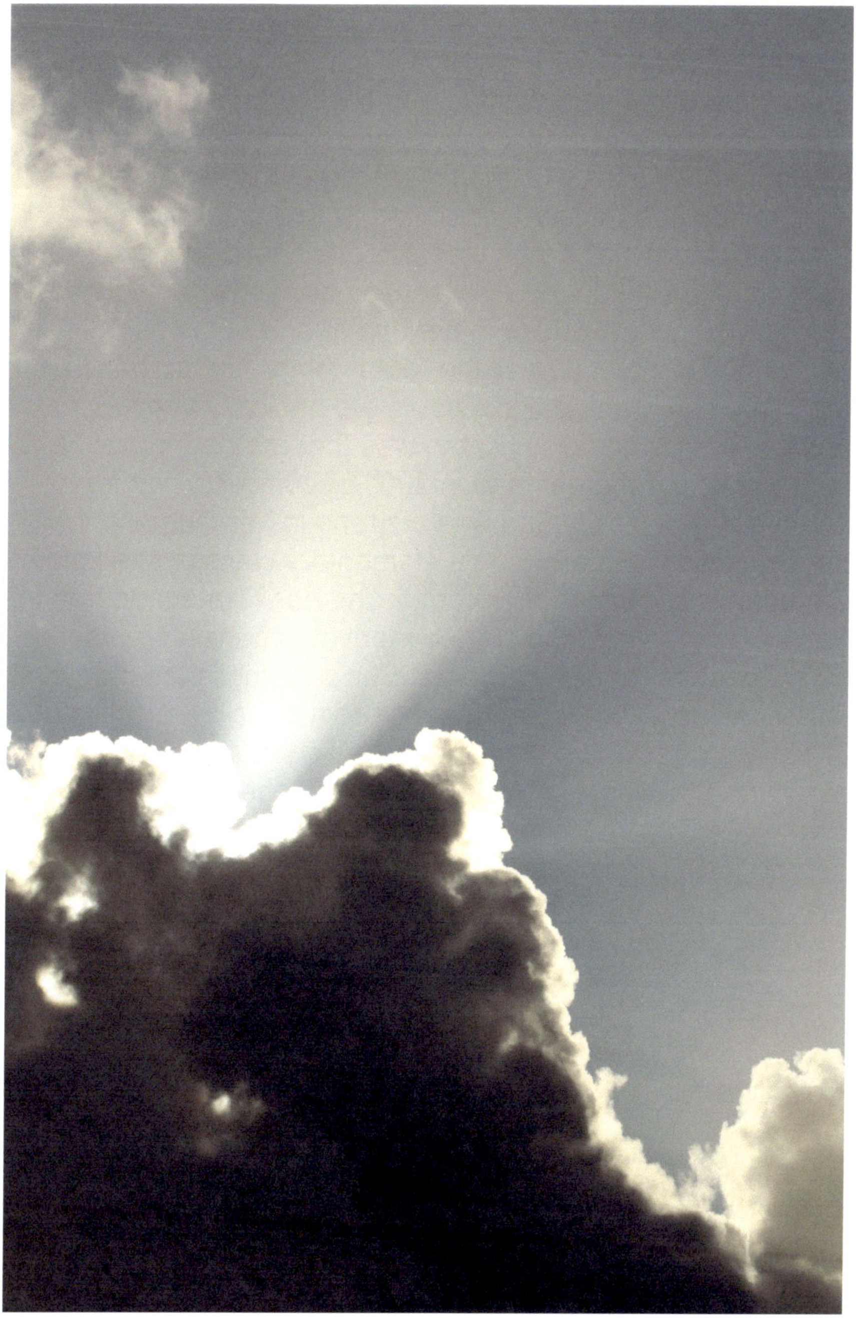

Karen's Story

This is the story of my sister Karen's battle with Inflammatory Breast Cancer. First, I want to share with you a few things about my sister's life prior to IBC. Karen was born on September 21, 1947, the first of three children. We were raised in a middle-income family in a small town in Southwest Virginia. Karen was a healthy child and adult. She had the usual childhood illnesses, an appendectomy when she was 18, and shingles in her eye at age 56. In her later adult life she tried to do all the "right" things for her health; for example, she drank bottled water, ate basically vegetables, and walked for exercise. Karen was the "mother" in our family after our mother died in 2001 of complications from Alzheimer's disease. She was a strong in her faith and in her convictions. Karen taught elementary classes at a local Christian school and, after completing her Masters degree in Family Counseling, she started a private counseling practice that was open for several years. She accomplished many things in her 58 years and met her goal of being successful in many careers. She has been a hair stylist, the county magistrate, a Mary Kay lady, a hospital secretary, and the owner of a Tea Room in our small hometown. The folks around town lovingly called her the "Tea Lady." Throughout her adult life her primary commitment was to God, her children, and her family.

Now, I want to tell you about Karen and IBC.

Symptoms

November 2004: On Thanksgiving day in 2004, Karen showed me a place on the lower right side of her right breast that was red, had a rash, and was warm and itchy. We agreed she needed to see her doctor immediately.

Initial diagnosis

December 2004: Karen saw her medical doctor, who treated her for mastitis for two rounds of antibiotics. Then she was seen by a surgeon who treated her with another round of antibiotics. Her son, who is a doctor of chiropractic medicine, said "enough" and scheduled a fine needle biopsy at a clinic in a nearby city where a diagnosis is given at the time of the biopsy.

Corrected Diagnosis

Karen and I went for the fine needle biopsy and she was told it was cancer. She was very calm about it, just planning what to do next. A trip to the surgeon followed. He did a core biopsy and port insertion and she was diagnosed with IBC.

January 2005: Appointment with oncologist with a PET scan and much blood work to follow. (The PET scan was clear except for the breast area and I believe some axillary lymph nodes. Her oncologist told us later that just because a PET scan shows clear doesn't mean the body is clear...that it takes billions of cancer cells to show a small area on the scan.)

Treatment

February/March 2005: Karen began chemotherapy with Adriamycin/Cytoxan, four treatments over a 12-week period. A medicine was also given to her to eliminate nausea. This was given two days before and the day of chemo. During this time Karen did not have nausea, just weakness. Her white blood cell count would drop and she incurred one hospital visit due to this. There also was a problem with her red blood cell count for which she received injections. Karen continued to work (she was now managing her son's chiropractic/

medical practice) except for the week of chemo. It seemed by the time the next chemo was due, she had just gotten back on her feet. Karen was always positive in her belief that she would conquer this disease. She had a strong faith in God.

April/May: Karen began Taxotere. She experienced nosebleeds, bleeding underneath her nails, and weakness, but she was still able to function and even do some of her work.

July 7, 2005: Karen completed the Taxotere regime and we were readying for her surgery, scheduled for August 1.

July 11, 2005: Karen was admitted to the hospital after an episode of inability to breathe. She was diagnosed with blood clots and pneumonia in her lungs.

July 28, 2005: Karen came home from the hospital.

July 29, 2005: Karen was re-admitted to the hospital with breathing difficulties.

August 1, 2005: A lung biopsy was done, which showed the cancer had metastasized to the lungs and was extensive in the chest cavity. The doctor said she had maybe three months left to live.

August 16, 2005: Karen came home from the hospital with hospice care. Even at this point, Karen did not believe she was going to die. She continued to have faith that she would be healed. She never signed the "do not resuscitate" instruction because I believe she thought it would show a lack of faith. (Her husband signed it later when she was admitted to the Hospice House.)

August/September: Karen had become very immobile,

was on oxygen all the time, and was very weak. She was taking morphine and Ativan. By this time, I was spending every day and some nights with her. She seemed comforted to know I was with her. We had always been very close, being only 20 months apart in age. Her children and husband as well as some dear friends assisted with her care but she wanted me listed as caregiver with the hospice. On Labor Day we had a family picnic. On September 21, we had a birthday party for her. She was so precious…always the gracious lady…always concerned with everyone's well-being. We had a wonderful party, but I know it stressed her body even though she did not say so. On September 22, she awoke at 4:00 am and said she was going to Hospice House…she was afraid and was going there, so the family should call and make the arrangements or she would. I believe she knew the end was near and she wanted to be at the Hospice House, where she would receive her pain medicine and Ativan without discussion. (Her son had tried to limit her medication because he wanted her to be lucid. His intentions were good but not reasonable, and they brought on a confrontation between us.) I gave her meds as the hospice ordered when I was with her. When families are so stressed in a situation of illness, the family members are not always going to agree. Her daughter and son made the arrangements for her to go to Hospice House and she and my daughter, Sarah, who is a nurse, rode there by ambulance. Her daughter, Sabrina, and I drove. We arrived at Hospice House and met with her oncologist, who answered all our questions as best she could. A lovely lady, the oncologist was so kind and caring. I asked Karen if she wanted me to stay and she said she knew it was too much to ask but she wanted me with her all the time. I told her I would go home and pack my bag, which I did, and I stayed with her until she passed away. During our time at Hospice House, we shared some precious times. She told me she was not afraid to die, that she knew where she was going…she just hated to leave everyone behind. She also said she was afraid of smothering. We spoke of Mother's death. After the oncologist's visit, I prayed with Karen, Sarah, and Sabrina, and Karen said, "Thank you for being so wise." I said, "You are the wise one, I'm the silly one." She said, "Hmmm….silly is joy!" Karen continued to worsen but seemed to hold on until my brother and his wife arrived from out of town on September 23. She so looked forward to their arrival and we had a sleepover at Hospice House that night and laughed and had a great time. She was so full of life and energy and love. She did not go to sleep until 1:30 am and was up at 6:10 am talking more. My brother left the next morning and she immediately began to decline. On September 27, Karen was very weak and was having difficulty breathing. This is when she surrendered her will to His and prayed if this is how it's going to be…let's move on. Visitors were many, family and friends, but she became silent.

October 4, 2005: My sweet sister, passed from this room to her Heavenly home at 1:30 am. Her childhood friend and I were holding her hands and her son was holding her. I believe that angels escorted her as she raised her arms toward heaven. The nurses at Hospice House said that they believed angels circled above all the time. So sweet…one man told me that he considered Hospice House the front porch of Heaven. Isn't that precious?

I learned so much from my sister during life and during her illness and death. Her faith, strength, and courage will be forever etched in the hearts of those who loved her. In October of 2006, I established the Karen Rasnick Bradley Annual Breast Cancer Awareness Program that I conducted at the local high school. I think Karen would be pleased to know education is being done in her memory and in honor of her life. I think it is important to get the word out about

Inflammatory Breast Cancer and the symptoms.

It has been one year and four months since my sister passed away and I miss her every day. It gives me great comfort to know she is probably smiling as I continue to find my way without her.

There are stories of hope and success with some IBC patients and I pray research continues and a cure is found. My sister fought a courageous battle with Inflammatory Breast Cancer that ended October 4, 2005, at age 58, only ten months after diagnosis. Her legacy of courage and hope lives on.

—Penelope Rasnick Hensley

Ed. Note: Penelope sat with her sister the night she passed and read to her. Here is what she read:

Quieted With His Love
by Tom Norvell
September 20, 2005

As I worked my way through some devotional readings, I came across this passage: "*The LORD your God is with you, he is mighty to save. He will take great delight in you, he will quiet you with his love, he will rejoice over you with singing.*" (Zephaniah 3:17)

I thought of my life. I thought of what the passage says about God and how He feels about me. He is mighty to save. He will take great delight in me. He will quiet me with his love. He will rejoice over me. I confess that although I do not know if I fully understand what it means to be quieted by His love, I do know that there is something inside me that says, "I need that, Lord!" As I pondered more, I prayed, "Lord, please quiet me with Your love."

"Lord, please quiet me with Your love.
"Lord, please quiet me with Your love.
"Lord, please quiet me with Your love."

"Lord, I get loud sometimes. Not so much verbally loud, but my spirit gets loud. My heart gets loud. My mind gets loud. The world around me gets loud and the loudness overwhelms me to the point that everything within me and around me seems to be loud. So, Lord, please quiet me with Your love.

"In these times of unrest and confusion in our nation and world, I need to be quieted by your love, dear Lord. Decisions are being made that may well change the way we live and function as a people. Lord, please quiet me with Your love.

"As the years pass more rapidly than my mind can comprehend, I need to be quieted with Your love. I cannot keep up. I try, but I seem to fall farther and farther behind. Lord, please quiet me with Your love.

"In times when I fear for my very life and for the lives of my family and friends, I need to be quieted by Your love. In times when my spirit in under attack by the Enemy to such an extent that I begin to wonder if You are still there, I need to be quieted by Your love. Lord, please quiet me with Your love.

"In times of discouragement when I have failed to live like You have asked me to live, I need to be quieted by Your love. In times of disappointment over dreams that have faded and when other people have failed to live up to my expectations, I need to be quieted by Your love. Lord, please quiet me with Your love.

"In times of loss and my heart has been broken, I need to

be quieted by your love. In times of sadness when a joyful spirit seems too much to consider, I need to be quieted by Your love. Lord, please quiet me with Your love.

"In times of suffering and pain as the result of another's actions or my own, I need to be quieted by Your love. In times when others are suffering because of my actions and I am helpless to undo what I have done, I need to be quieted by Your love. And they need to be quieted by Your love. Lord, please quiet me with Your love.

"In times of distress and anxiety over all that I must do, or feel that I must do, I need to be quieted by Your love. In times when life is so loud that I cannot hear my own thoughts, I need to be quieted by Your love. Lord, please quiet me with Your love.

"Unless You quiet me with Your love, dear Lord, my life will surely be filled with noises that may drown Your voice from my ears. Lord, I need to be quieted by Your love.

"When I remind myself that You are with me, when I contemplate Your power, when I consider that You take great delight in me and when I think of You rejoicing over me with singing because of Your love for me, I am quieted. My heart is quieted. My spirit rests.

"Lord, You have quieted me with Your love."

The LORD your God is with you, he is mighty to save. He will take great delight in you, he will quiet you with his love, he will rejoice over you with singing. (Zephaniah 3:17)

Ed. Note: As Penelope mentioned, Karen passed away on October 4, 2005. She was 58.

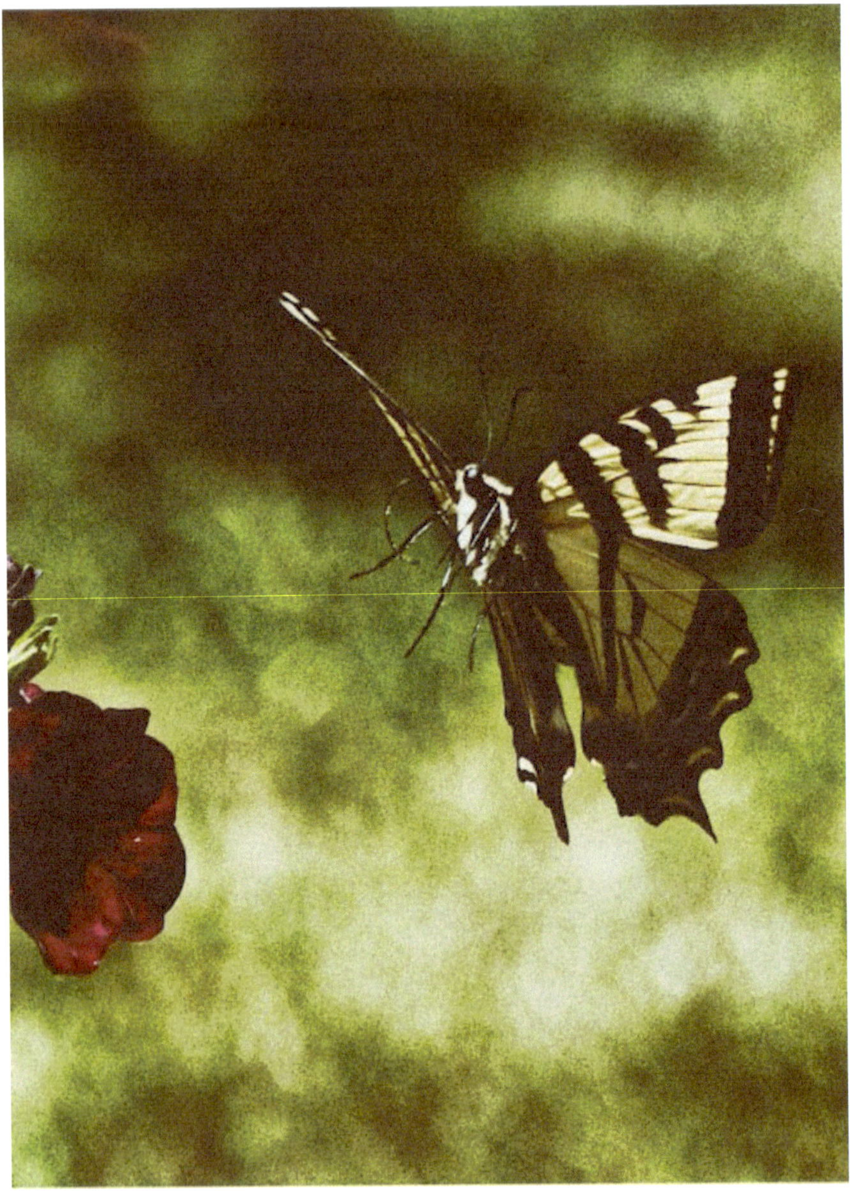

Sandra's Story

Men occasionally stumble over the truth,
but most of them pick themselves up and
hurry off as if nothing ever happened.
Sir Winston Churchill

Symptoms

I started having symptoms in July 2002. I had terrible pain in my left breast but after a month, the pain wasn't so bad. I put this down to the fact that I was in menopause and left it. I had another period and my breast swelled up even more and I had terrific pain. The pain was so bad I had to hold my breast in my hand as I walked. My skin became peau d'orange, my nipple was inverted, and my breast misshapen. In October I discovered a mass at the 6 o'clock position on my breast that was very painful to the touch. I was terrified as my mother, two aunts, and two first cousins had all died of breast cancer before age 55 and one of my cousins had ovarian cancer at the same time as breast cancer.

Diagnosis

I finally went to see my primary physician, a general practitioner, who wasn't convinced that there was anything seriously wrong but decided to send me to see a surgeon as I was so anxious about my family history. Two days later I saw the consultant physician. My breast was so swollen that when they took the mammogram, he couldn't see anything for the inflammation inside the breast. He said that the lymph nodes were affected as was a lymph node in the neck. He told me that although they couldn't see anything, that I definitely had breast cancer and that "it wasn't in the early stages." I was devastated, especially in the light of my mother's history. I cried really deeply and was in total shock. I couldn't stop crying, so the surgeon sent me out to speak with the breast care nurse, who was very supportive. My main thought at the time was how I was going to tell my daughter. The surgeon gave me an appointment for a biopsy in two days and when I got outside I collapsed. When we got home my husband broke down crying.

My daughter, Beth, was due down that weekend anyway as we were going to a rugby match. She seemed quite calm when we met her at the train, but when we all sat down in the restaurant she broke down in tears. On Saturday Beth and I went to the rugby match. It did me a world of good because I felt I let a lot of anger out.

Treatment

I turned up at the hospital two days later and had the biopsy and went back in to see the consultant surgeon. By now the skin underneath my breast was changing colour. He told me that my condition was serious (he didn't tell me what it was called) and said he was sending me to the Velindre Cancer Centre in Cardiff to see someone who specializes in a treatment where I would be given chemotherapy, and after three sessions, if the tumor had shrunk, they would operate. I then saw a consultant oncologist, who told me I had IBC and that it was Stage III, Grade III. He told me I would be started on chemotherapy. After the three sessions, I had a scan which revealed that the tumour had gone. My lymph nodes under my arm and in my neck were normal.

That was February 2003. I had to continue with the chemotherapy, spending some time in hospital, suffering an infection and having a blood transfusion. During that time I also had severe bouts of diarrhea and sickness, and I lost all my hair and eye lashes and eye brows (as you do) and had a kidney stone. My teeth started breaking and my mouth was full of ulcers. I found a lump in my mouth that was a suspect tumor but it turned out not to be. After the sixth session, I saw my oncologist, who told me that he was not going to do a mastectomy. I still have both breasts. It is nearly four years since my diagnosis and I feel great. Because of the way the IBC went, the treatment I received means that I get the same symptoms at regular intervals that I had with IBC: swollen breasts, redness, areola turning yellow, and pain. I still get scared but I know that that's ok.

I have seen my oncologist and the surgeon several times since and they both said that what happened to me was "fantastic and amazing." What I'm saying here is NEVER GIVE UP HOPE. The reason I say this is that just after I was diagnosed, a breast cancer nurse came to my house to explain the gory details of my disease to me and I was distraught when she left. She insisted that I would be having a mastectomy "because everyone with this disease does" and I was no different and I had better get used to it. Within ten minutes of her going I felt a surge of energy and hope rush through my body and I said to my husband, "How dare she say how this disease is going to turn out. I will not let her do that." That surge of energy (whatever it was) lasted for about an hour and from that moment on, I was on a mission to survive.

I got in touch with a Spiritual Healing Centre (by letter) and they said prayers for me and that comforted me a lot. I talked to my breast every day and got angry with it and told it that it had to get better, that I couldn't allow it to do this yet again in my family. A psychologist friend of mine introduced me to Bernie Siegel, MD, and I read his books and was uplifted. Nothing was stopping me now! And then I had a setback. The same friend loaned me a book about IBC and I read about IBC for the first time. I stayed up all night crying.

But the following day, I told myself that it couldn't happen to me. I wasn't going to die. I said it out loud every day. Every time I said it I became more energetic. Each time I had chemo I was sick for the first ten days, but the rest of the time until the next session, I lived it up and did everything I wanted to do.

At the beginning of the illness I had been to see *Lord of the Rings*, and when I was ill in the beginning and really down, my husband put Frodo Baggins picture into a frame and put it at the side of the bed and told me that I was going on a journey and had to be brave like Frodo, that family and friends were willing me to get well and also relying on me to lead the way and they would follow. That picture is now hanging up in the kitchen!

I have seen my oncologist several times since and he said he had not seen anything like this. A tumour disappearing happens only in about five percent of cases (and that includes other types of breast cancer). I then had radiotherapy to my breast and neck and to an internal site through my back. My oncologist told me that it was the most radiotherapy that a person could take. When I was being "measured up" for the treatment, my oncologist was at Heathrow Airport just arriving back from a conference in the US. He wanted to ensure that everything was being done properly and phoned on his mobile and stayed on it. His assistant had to speak to him on the phone relaying every move until he was satisfied! Radiotherapy was the easiest of the treatments. I went for treatment every day for five weeks, 25 miles there and 25 miles back.

When I finished radiotherapy I went back to my primary physician to tell him that I had finished at the hospital, and he told me that because he had never heard of IBC, he had looked it up on the computer, and he asked me if I wanted tranquillizers to get me through the next few months. I started to cry and told him that my oncologist had said the tumour had gone. He then said, "They will tell you that, but the reality of the situation is that you are not going to survive." He then told me that it was no use crying and that if I took tranquillizers it would help until the time arrived. He said that everyone in my position went on tranquillizers and if I changed my mind, then I was to go back to him. This week I had great satisfaction of giving an interview to our local paper and telling them about IBC and my run-in with it. I hope he reads it. I should have been dead three years ago according to him!

Apart from the fact that I had IBC, I've also been told by the Genetics Department that I am at high risk for the breast cancer gene. My daughter and I decided not to go for the test as we are both being monitored and I didn't want that hanging over our heads.

One year after the tumor disappeared I broke my wrist! I have some autoimmune disease of the mouth as a result of the treatment I've had, which has left me with continuous patches of ulcers. I don't care about that. It was only three months ago that my oncologist told me that if the chemo hadn't got rid of the tumour, I would have been "in big trouble."

The only drug I'm taking now is Tamoxifen, which I started when radiotherapy finished. Next year I will be going on Femara.

I am a vegetarian, I take lots of vitamins and supplements and have taken up drumming.

Never give up hope, girls. Hope is the magic thing in our lives. Hope can move mountains and can bring about miracles. Don't ever, ever give up. We can beat this thing.

I'm sorry this was so long. I have been uneasy about telling my story because I know you are all going through so much and I didn't want to seem flippant. I hope I haven't done that.

I think about you all every day and remember you in my prayers.

Everyone told me that what happened to me couldn't be done, but I have come this far. You can too.

Ed. Note: No followup information is available on Sandra.

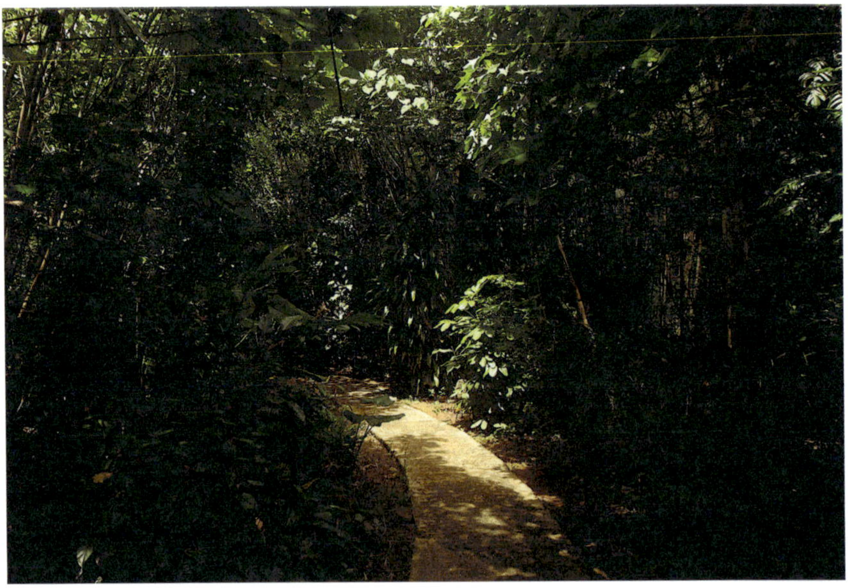

Rich & Doracina's Story

Do not go where the path may lead, go instead where there is no path and leave a trail.
Ralph Waldo Emerson

In 1969 I came home from the military. I wasn't home for very long before I noticed a young woman living with her relatives just next door. The sister she lived with was from Brasil (that is how Brazilians spell it) and Doracina had come to be with her. My first attempt at making contact was quite a flop in that she did not speak any English, and I spoke absolutely no Portuguese. As luck had it, one evening I noticed her walking home with a book under her arm. I got her attention with a remark about the weather and asked what she was reading. She was taking English as a second language in our local church. I offered to help with her studies (pretty slick, ay?) and that was the start of the rest of my life. Looking back, I think I learned more Portuguese than she learned English, but so what.

Doracina was the youngest of 15 children—including three sets of twins. Her family lived on a ranch in southern Brasil. Each child in the family had a job to do. Her job was to mount a horse each day and ride out with her father to bring in the cows. On one of our visits to her family, I had the thrill of seeing just how well she could ride a horse. I was so proud of her skills.

Doracina had a pretty uneventful medical history prior to her first pregnancy, which came a year after our 1971 marriage. We lost a child to a spontaneous miscarriage. She was treated for anemia by our family doctor. A year after the miscarriage our son Roger was born via Cesarean section. She did not breast feed the baby. Until September 2000, that was the extent of her medical history.

For almost 30 years our life was normal, or as normal as can be expected for two people from completely different cultures and languages. "What language did you speak at home?" is an often asked question. Thinking back I have to honestly say, "I don't know." Roger grew up fluent in both English and Portuguese, so I guess it was both. Doracina was always shy about her English and always looked toward me to talk. However, because Portuguese and Spanish are quite similar and because of the heavy Spanish-speaking population in our area, she mastered Spanish. We had gone to a wedding of a Mexican couple once, and I was so proud of her ability to converse with all the guests.

Symptoms

In August of 2000 I noticed that her left arm was a bit swollen. I asked whether she had been bitten by a bug. She could not find any other marks on the arm and dismissed it as a slight infection "or something." I told her that we would give it a week to get better and then go to a doctor. She was never one for doctors and we did not have one in the area. The last doctor we had been to was in Clifton, NJ. So, in anticipation of going for a penicillin shot, I set out to find a doctor, hoping that I could use the "infected" area as an excuse to get her going on a regular schedule of general checkups. I checked the area for a doctor that she could communicate with. My two main objectives that it be a female internist and one who spoke Spanish. I found such a doctor in the town of Dover, NJ, a few miles from us.

After a week of continued swelling, I called the doctor and asked to get in as soon as possible, fearing that the "infection" would only worsen. We were in the doctor's office the next day, August 22. Our doctor was a young intelligent Columbian woman who Doracina took to right away. As she did her exam she spoke with both of us, mostly in Spanish, but to be sure I understood she switched often to English. She did a quick check and then did a breast exam. On completion, she said, "I want Doracina to get a mammogram and ultra-sound of the left breast right away. I agreed but asked what she thought of the arm swelling. That was why we were there. She said "Well, I cannot find any lumps there but I think that is the problem. I think she has breast cancer." My first reaction was that this beautiful young woman was way off base. How long will it be before we get some antibiotics into that arm? After all, even she said there is no lump and we all know that women with breast cancer have a lump. Don't they? Our doctor called the hospital herself and arranged for us to be there the next day. I was to learn later on that our doctor was quite an exception and that her instant diagnosis of IBC was not the norm. Women are constantly misdiagnosed and treated for weeks, even months, with antibiotics. Much as we didn't want to hear "cancer," we had no time to fool around and I am grateful to our doctor for her skill and ability.

The radiologist came to me saying that there were no lumps in either breast but there was something "suspicions" in the left breast that our doctor might want us to test further. We left the hospital thinking that this thing was going a bit too far. By 2 pm that afternoon, our doctor called me. She wanted us to go to a surgeon and have a biopsy done on the left breast. She gave me the name of a surgeon in the area, and I called. Three days later we walked into the Same Day Surgery Unit of St. Clare's Hospital in Dover, after having the pre-surgery testing the day before.

We went right into the prep room, and they took her vitals and got a line started. I was led out to the waiting room and I sat with family members of other patients. I sat there for about four hours, enough time to convince myself that we were going through all this for nothing. The doctor finally came out with a very serious face. He sat down with me and said that she was OK but that she did indeed have cancer. "It's an inflammatory cancer." That was the first time I'd ever heard about IBC and to tell you the truth, it didn't mean anything to me. I had read about Invasive Ductal Carcinoma and Lobular Carcinoma and all I could find in the few days I had to look for information. Nothing I read mentioned inflammatory so I figured he was just talking about the inflammation in her arm.

When they called me in, she was sitting in one of those lounge chairs. I had to be the one to tell her that she had breast cancer. She was confused. She asked how could that be. "I don't eat anything bad and I take care of myself. Maybe it's just a small cancer, and they can take care of it," she said. Filled with doubt, fear, confusion and denial, I took my wife home, not knowing what lay ahead of us. We were home for less than an hour when our doctor called.

"Rich, I want you to get her into treatment as soon as possible. This week. She has a very dangerous form of cancer, and it must be treated aggressively." Well, how the heck could this be? Everybody I ever heard of who had breast cancer went to the doctor, "caught it in time," and then took their time going over treatment options. What the heck did we do wrong?

My next call was to Sloan Kettering who had a facility right there in Denville, NJ, 20 miles from our home. Before she even took my name, the scheduler at Sloan asked, "What insurance do you have?" I had Aetna at the time. I was told that I would have to foot all the money for treatment up front, and any insurance payments were between me and my insurance company. My company was self-insured, and the company dictated the rules of payment to the insurance company. I knew that their coverage would have left me responsible for 90% of Sloan's bills.

Our doctor said to hurry up so I started checking available oncologists in the area and found one.

The day of the appointment, the oncologist came into the room with all the reports in his arms. As he slipped the films into the viewer on the wall he said to us, "You know, we have a very serious situation here." He did his exam, found nothing that he hadn't expected, and went over the treatment plan and all of our questions. I tried to get him to give an indication of just what kind of treatment time we were looking at. His only response, and I will respect him for it always, was, "I never tell a person how long they have. We are going to do all we can to keep Doracina alive and active for as long as we can." So there it was: We are not curing this. We will never see the end of cancer until cancer sees the end of us. Thus began the fight for Doracina's life. For our life.

Treatment

The first offensive: CAF (Cytoxan, Andriamycin and 5FU) we were told would be once every three weeks, and the first open battle took place that following Tuesday at the oncologist's Denville office.

I had never seen my wife so sick. In my twenty years of EMT work I had rarely seen people that sick. Within a week she was almost a complete invalid. She could not eat or stop vomiting. She was too weak to walk across the house without stopping for a rest. We still had to get a portacath put in, and I was worried that this simple procedure would be too much for her. She did, however, manage to get through it.

I searched the Internet for all I could about this monster that was attacking our life. The best I could find was on the American Cancer Society site. They stated, "Inflammatory Breast Cancer is a very aggressive form off the disease and the prognosis is usually very poor." That was about it.

It was a month, and I still did not have a name for this disease. It was inflammatory, but what was it? Our doctor told me that was the name of the disease: Inflammatory Breast Cancer. All along I thought they were referring to the appearance of the skin which had turned angry red and had the orange peel appearance. “Just search for Inflammatory Breast Cancer, Rich. You should be able to find something.”

I went to the computer the next day and looked up IBC. I went right to an IBC help page, www.ibcsupport.org, that was created by Pete Bevin and Menya Wolfe. IBC is a killer. There was, however, on that site a link to the IBC Support mailing list. I signed up and found a world of information, love, and support from so many others fighting IBC. The group became part of our life and still is part of mine. With the IBC Support group, we were not alone. We had a family of love.

After three treatments, the oncologist determined that a drop in dosage was called for. This did help a bit, but by the end of her sixth treatment a multigated acquisition (MUGA) scan[5] showed that her cardiac output was dropping too low, and the “A” in the CAF chemotherapy was replaced by “M”: Methotrexate. CMF. This drug was used for 21 treatments.

So, we were into the fray. Chemotherapy became part of our life. Side effects were severe. Her blood count would plummet, and I was giving her Lukin and Procrit shots all the time. The edema in her left arm was limiting my sites for injections, but I was soon to learn that these were the good times when it came to places for a shot. Two legs and the right arm. Soon, my target area would be severely limited.

---

5 A multigated acquisition (MUGA) scan creates video images of the ventricles (lower chambers of the heart that hold blood) to check whether they are pumping blood properly. It can identify chemotherapy-related heart damage.

In January of 2001 Doracina's right leg swelled and became hot to the touch. I might have missed the IBC diagnosis, but I surely knew a blood clot when I saw it. The oncologist sent us right to the hospital for a Doppler study. We spent 20 days in the hospital this time.

The drug mix that seemed to do the best for us, CMF, finally lost its ability to hold back the cancer. The IBC monster was on the march again and in May of 2002 we were switched to weekly Taxol infusions. Taxol had its own set of chemo reactions and Doracina braced herself. By this time, she was the picture of a chronically ill person. She was weak and both legs were 1.5 to 2 times their normal size from the edema caused by the clot in the IVC filter. She took to sleeping quite a bit during the day. She would get up and watch the Mass on TV. Thank God for EWTN (the Catholic television network). She could always tune in to hear her Mass or listen to priests talk about the world we live in. Doracina's faith was unshakable. She took all the suffering as part of life and prayed constantly, if not for a cure then for the strength to endure. Whenever she had a problem she would not tell me because she didn't want to complain, but just report it in case there was something we could do about it.

I am not too sure just how well the Taxol worked. Her overall general condition was steadily declining so much that it was hard to tell. During Taxol we had a few bouts with recurring cellulitis, mostly in the left arm that was constantly swollen. Antibiotics were given and they worked. One, Levaquin, worked really well but took a toll on Doracina, as it really made her sick.

Dr. Adler used tumor markers, along with Doracina's presentation at each weekly visit, to determine the chemo's ability to help. Once tumor markers went down, he would order a new set of bone and CT scans as he changed drugs.

This happened every two to three months.

She became so weak that I used to dread those days in the hospital almost as much as she did. At least we were fortunate in that the oncologist always had the reports faxed to him and would call us that afternoon to let us know. Each time he gave us some encouragement. Yet, each time, there was something bad. I learned to hate the word "uptake."

By November of 2002, any good that the Taxol was doing weakened. CT and bone scans showed that the disease was again taking off. Not only that, skin mets[6] had started to make their appearance. Big ugly ulcers starting on her left breast. The drug of choice this time was Navelbine every two weeks. As for side effects, Doracina did well on Navelbine but by now her condition was so weakened that she could never have tolerated the big guns of CAF. Navelbine had to work. At the beginning of her treatment, I had asked the oncologist what we would do if the CAF didn't work. He told me that he would switch to something else. "This disease is evasive, but we have plenty of tricks up our sleeves too." I was beginning to fear that he was running out of tricks.

Treatment changes

Navelbine was beginning to fail. Doracina was weakening. In May what seemed to be a controlled downhill slide turned into an uncontrollable race to a crash. It started with the discovery of fluid in the pleural space of her right lung. A thoracentesis removed almost two liters of fluid. The oncologist gave up on Navelbine and we went onto Gemzar, supposedly a treatment a week for three weeks and then a week off. We never managed to finish one series of this treatment. The first week of June found us in the hospital

6 Skin metastases refer to the growth of cancer cells in the skin originating from an internal cancer.

again with a thoracentesis needed on the left lung. Because the right side was filled with fluid again and had filled so fast, a pleurodesis was recommended for that side. We were in the hospital for six days this time. Unlike the thoracentesis, the pleurodesis is a painful process. The insertion of a catheter was followed by four days lying still while a pump at the side of the bed drained the area. Thank God they let me stay with her. Between the pump on one side of the bed and the IV on the other hooked up to her port, the poor woman was being tortured. She couldn't even find the buzzer at the side of her bed half of the time. She had only my voice to ask for the morphine that was ordered every four hours. She couldn't even turn in bed, let alone make it to the bathroom.

We returned from that trip to the hospital at an all time low. The next week, on June 1, we had an appointment with the oncologist for another try at Gemzar. Doracina just barely made it to the office. She wore her slippers. She never went out in her slippers, always insisting on my getting at least her soft sneakers on over her swollen feet. I somehow knew that our days of aggressive treatment were over and tried to prepare her for it on the trip to Denville. I told her that we might want to skip this treatment and wait a while. We sat with the oncologist . He did a short exam, checked her blood work, and said, "Well, your blood work is OK for a treatment, but what about you?" Doracina told him she felt weak and tired from the hospital stay.

He closed her file, dropped it on his desk as if in defeat, and said, "Well, I can see no sense in continuing with this chemo. It is causing more harm than good. We'd better concentrate on comfort care." Doracina understood what was being said. She looked up at me and said in Portuguese, "Ask him if we can just rest for a month or two and maybe when I get my strength back we can try chemo again." I turned to the doctor and translated. He hesitated;

he was not a man to lie to a patient, but neither could he crush this woman. We had been together for three years. He ran to the hospital at night when we had problems. He heard all our pains. He looked up at me as if silently pleading with me for the right words. He said "*Yes, sure. I can go along with that. Let's just not make any appointments right now. But, I do want you to find a hospice that you feel comfortable with to get this pain under control and I will work with them in whatever is needed.*"

My mission had changed. I now had to find a hospice. Hospice care, I soon found out, is not just a place to die. They are there to help a person live in dignity and be as comfortable as possible when they reach the end of life.

After I left Doracina at home, I went to the hospice unit in Dover, NJ. They rent a ten-room wing from St. Clare's Hospital. Thus began our last and most difficult period. The oncologist prescribed Oxycontin 20 mg. twice a day. This soon became ineffective, and we worked our way up to 100 mg. Doracina began to sleep more and more. She could not eat. Sometime in June of 2003 her abdomen began to distend. It was hard and painful. She had been suffering from an old adversary that had plagued her since the Navelbine days: constipation.

One Sunday Doracina lay there almost defeated. I offered to call the doctor and try to take her to the hospital for a paracentesis, a simple procedure to remove the fluid from the abdomen. Doracina agreed and I called the oncologist's office, spoke with his covering doctor, and told him that we needed to get this done today. The doctor, who recommended that we wait until Monday morning and go down to the office first, agreed to call ahead to the ER. I insisted that we needed this procedure right away.

She spent the afternoon and evening in that ER. After one

ten-minute check by the ER doctor, she was left on a hard ER stretcher for hours. I was trying to get something for her pain. Finally, they ordered that the port be accessed and she be given morphine. After three years of constant use, her port had nearly had it. They called down a nurse practitioner to access the port. Three sticks later she thought she had it, and they started the morphine drip. That night we found out that it was a miss and no drug ever got into Doracina's veins.

After all this waiting, the ER doctor came in and told us that they had to do the procedure under ultra sound in radiology the next morning. Our doctor had arranged that Doracina be admitted for the night so that she could be monitored. So, back up to the oncology unit on the second floor for our last night in the hospital. As soon as we entered the room, I asked the oncology nurse to check the port access as it did not seem to be functioning. She checked and confirmed my suspicion. She re-accessed the port and after ten hours with no pain medication, Doracina finally rested a bit.

The next morning the oncologist's partner came in. He confirmed that we would be in radiology in an hour or two. I sat and talked to him about this pain management. We could not get it under control. I was lost. How much longer was she to suffer? I asked about going to the hospice in Dover. He told me that he would get the process going and that we could go right from the hospital to Dover. We decided that this would be a temporary thing only to get the pain under control. Then she was wheeled down to radiology for what we thought would be a paracentesis under ultra-sound. When we got there the tech ran the instrument over Doracina's abdomen. She told me that she didn't think there was any fluid there. The doctor came in and confirmed it. So, of course, I insisted, "Then what is blowing her belly up like that? Pregnancy?"

It was tumors. They were growing and had taken over her entire abdomen, choking the life out of my wife from within, attacking one organ after another, one system after another. Three years prior, our doctor told me to prepare for this. A few weeks ago, the oncologist told me to go to hospice care. That very morning, I asked the oncologist's partner point blank how much longer we had. His reply was, "It could be weeks, it could be months, but no more than three months." Still, I don't believe I had really heard any of them until now. As the radiologist looked at me and said that he could do nothing, I finally knew. Doracina was dying. She looked up at me as I wheeled her back to the room. I told her we were going to a "different" hospital. "St. Clare's in Dover has a unit that is just to help with pain. They will help us." I met with the hospice representative, signed all the papers, and Roger and I got Doracina into the car for the ten-minute ride to Dover.

Sometime during our first year of chemo Doracina took to eating a chicken sandwich from one of the fast food places on the way home. She always had a hard time swallowing pills so she would take her sandwich home and use it to disguise the pills she needed to take that morning. I bought her one, but after half an hour, she gave up trying to eat it. She couldn't even get a bite of it down. The tumors had taken so much space that nothing would go down.

Our arrival at the hospice was uneventful. The facility was clean, quiet, and very well-appointed. It was made to look as close to home and as far from a hospital as possible. Her private room was large and had a sofa bed for family. There was a big picture window with a view of a green hill. Everyone there was dedicated to the patients. We even joked about the room being like a hotel room and that we were on the second honeymoon that we had never taken. Roger, who lived in New Brunswick—about 65 miles away, came often and sat with us at night.

Although we could have stayed there, Doracina wanted to go home. After a week, we headed for home under the hospice care to begin our vigil. It was obvious now that I could no longer leave her alone.

Her sleep was so sporadic that I never knew when she would get up to go to the bathroom. Because of the meds, or just because of her independent ways, she would never call me. She would just try to get up. I did not lie in the bed for fear that I might fall into a deep sleep and miss her movement. I lived for Friday nights. At least at 5 pm on Friday I had no obligation to the world. I could be with Doracina until 8 am Monday morning. The weekends were as much hell for her as the weekdays but at least I could be there to share them with her.

Her skin mets by this time had gone wild. She had three big lesions on her breast, which I cleaned and dressed twice a day. Her sides and back had smaller, closed lesions. They itched badly.

Doracina's sleep became almost constant. One thing did happen four days before her death that, in hindsight, I think signaled that the end was upon us. I noticed that the edema in her legs and even her arm seemed to be going down. She was not taking in any fluid; the tumors had probably receded enough to allow her bowels to function. She became unresponsive and her breathing, not a problem until now, became shallow. She was going into shock. The fluid in her arms and legs was being called on by her trunk in the body's natural reaction to try to save the vital organs.

Doracina was always a fanatic about wearing her wedding ring. She would never leave the house without it. In her final months, she never could get that ring on. However, as the fluid left her arms, her hands became young again, like a teenager's. It was as if she knew what was coming and wanted to be sure she could have her ring on for all the world to see.

Not wanting to see her die struggling for air and noting that she needed to be suctioned, I called the hospice nurse. I told her we needed oxygen and a suction machine. She came right over and told me that it would be best for Doracina if we got her back into the Dover unit. That morning we were back at the hospice unit. Doracina was peaceful and resting as only those wonderful women at the hospice could make her. I sat next to her bed, watching her breath. Slower, then a lapse, then a few breaths. At around 3:00 pm she breathed no longer. I just waited. The nurse came in and checked Doracina. Then she got on one knee and took my hand, "It's over Rich...."

Ed. Note: Doracina passed away on August 19, 2003.

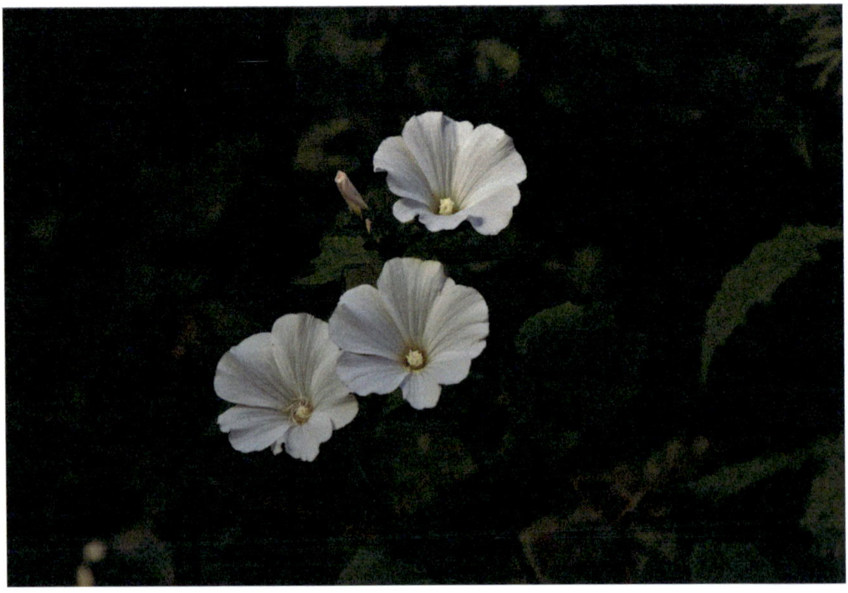

Kim's Story

There are three kinds of men. The one that learns by reading. The few who learn by observation. The rest of them have to pee on the electric fence for themselves.
Will Rogers

I was 48 years old, healthy and newly divorced, and blissfully happy. I had ridden horses all of my life and had just purchased a lovely dressage gelding who was imported from Holland last year, a horse of a lifetime, and we were anticipating the forthcoming '07 show season planning to be prepared and fit.

Not. That was July. On September 11 (ironically enough), I was talking to my coach and felt a sharp stabbing pain in my right breast. It was swollen like crazy and hot as hell. For a minute I attributed it to the underwire bra I wear to ride and thought to myself that I needed to invest in some better undergarments.

The next morning I had the good sense to call my friend Beth who is also a rider and a nurse of the highest order. I told her about the pain and she sent me to her friend who was a nurse practitioner for an OB/GYN. I got an appointment for October 2 (not mentioning that I had this problem, but just telling her that I needed my annual checkup). After the appointment, she immediately sent me to the Nashville Breast Center and I got an appointment with another nurse practitioner, who immediately called a surgeon.

Initial treatment

What a difference a few days makes. The surgeon gave me one week of antibiotics (there was no redness or skin changes at that time, just pain and swelling) and was not satisfied with the results. She ordered a mammogram, an ultrasound just to begin diagnostics, and quietly asked me if I had ever heard of IBC. She told me that I needed to have a biopsy because I might have it.

I was shocked. I don't have to describe the feeling to all of you who know...my life was perfect and then instantly upside down. I was furious.

Diagnosis

The following night, after hours, the surgeon called me to confirm that my nightmare was beginning. The results were back. I had IBC. Next step was CT/PET scans to determine whether there was metastasis and to have a port put in. A PORT. Good LORD. I felt like a candle that was melting. I could not breathe. I could not eat. Scream. Cry. I just sat there and tried to get a grip on myself. I don't think I ever did.

The following night was a consultation after hours with the surgeon . Fortunately I have a number of very dear friends, and Nancy was with me that night. I could not ask questions, nor think lucidly, let alone try to DRIVE the 35 miles from Gallatin to Nashville. It was a surreal visit and at that point I was still pretty sure it was not happening to me.

It couldn't be. I had a horse show to ride in Saturday. But it was. On Friday I got my first piece of good news. It looks like CT/PET scans showed that the cancer had not metastasized, save for one lymph node under the arm, and one spot on the skin, which by now was already growing a very "in-your-face-type" rash.

On Monday I had another surreal experience: the first oncology visit. It was as weird as the one with the surgeon. Again, I was totally incapable of a sensible thought. This time, however, I was armed with not only Nancy, but Beth, who took copious notes and made sense of them to me later, and my dear friend and dressage coach, Lynne. Bless my friends. There are no words.

The following morning I had the port put in. Chemo was to start on Friday, the 27th of October. Somehow between that Tuesday and Friday I found my faith...or, should I say, my faith once again found me. I decided if this cancer was gonna kill me, it was gonna have to work at it.

Game On. I welcomed the chemo like a long-lost friend and could almost feel the war inside my body as my breast shrunk in size and the pain subsided.

Treatment

So far I have managed the chemo fine. So far. I am learning to do the mouth wash thing, eating little meals, drinking lots of fluids, and forcing myself to rest. My chemo regimen is: Adriamycin and Cytoxan—four doses every two weeks, then weekly doses of Taxol and Herceptin for 12 weeks. Then I'll have surgery—I think that is gonna be tough—then radiation.

Then, the Tennessean Dressage show, where my partner, Nick, and I will compete in second level. By God or by Gosh, I have managed to keep riding and managing my business—just a little more slowly. But I'm two weeks into chemo and the panic is trying to set in.

That's where all of you come in, eh? Bless all of you who have already responded to my cry for help. Bless all of you who will become my sisters through a journey that, for a while, I thought only I was on. I can already tell that you will be life savers. I look forward to being able to reciprocate in the future.

Am I a Warrior yet?

Ed. Note: Kim is maintaining an active life as of this writing.

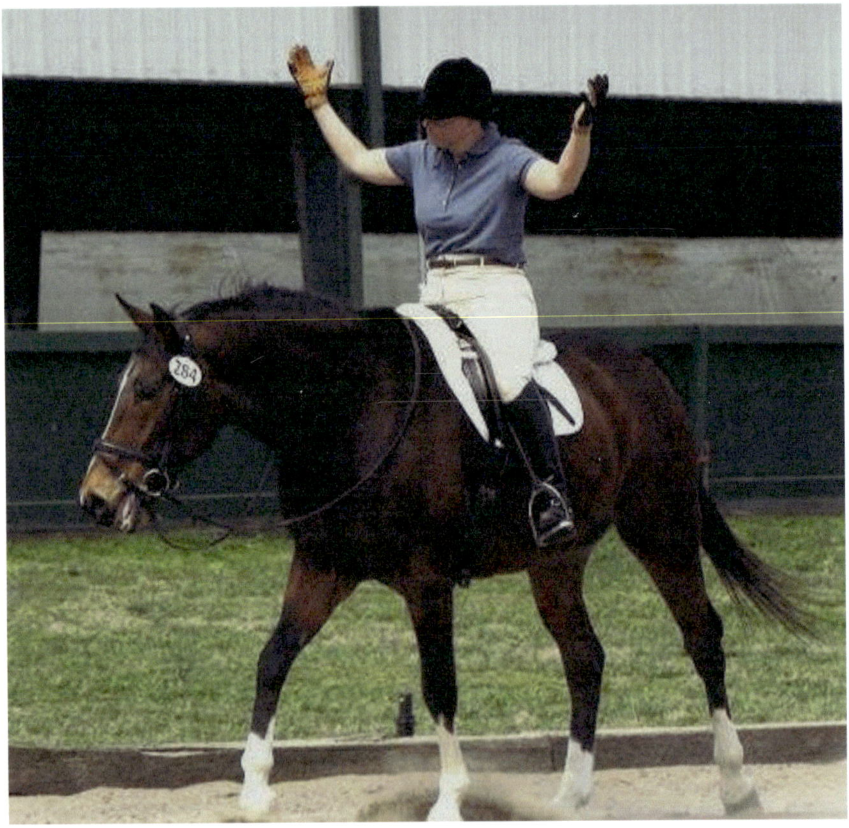

"Nick carried me when I couldn't carry myself."
Kim Alexander, NED (No Expiration Date)

Debbie's Story

I live in Halifax, Nova Scotia, Canada and have since I was born in March 1965. I went to Dalhousie University here in Halifax for my undergraduate degree, my medical degree and my family medicine residency. Up until the date of my diagnosis, I was working as a physician, most recently as a physician psychotherapist at the Centre for Emotions and Health here at Dalhousie University and the Capital District Mental Health Program (CDHMP). I also was the Team Leader for the GPs (General Practitioners) and GPPs (General Practitioners in Psychiatry) in the CDMHP, and the liaison between the Family Medicine and Psychiatric Departments at Dalhousie University. Prior to starting this multifaceted job in November 2003, I worked as a Private Family Practitioner since October 1998. Prior to that, I worked in the Canadian Military as a Military Physician (from October 1994 to October 1998). In that job, I was trained as a flight surgeon, a diving medical officer and I worked as the Senior Medical Officer at Shearwater Air Force Base. I also worked with the teams of people who helped in the aftermath of the crash of Swiss Air Flight 111 on September 3, 1998.

Symptoms

When I look back, I realize that I had vague suspicions of something "not quite right" in my left breast in December 2005, but thought that I was just experiencing discomfort due to a years-long history of "fibrocystic" breast tissue. I had a Pap test in January 2006, with a breast exam that was felt to be normal for me. In February I booked my first mammogram, which was scheduled for August due to the fact that it was supposed to be a screening exam and the usual routine is there's a long wait for those. I went to Yoga, without much trouble. In March, I noticed some more aching in my breast, which came to a head the night before we

(Jamie and I) went on a vacation to the Dominican Republic at the end of March. I noticed sharp pains in my left breast when I was lying on my chest getting a massage. Since we were due to leave early the next morning, I figured I'd have it checked out when we came back.

On our trip, my left breast began to swell dramatically, with what looked like a sunburn on the side near my armpit that my bikini top didn't cover. By the time we returned form the trip, the breast was hard, swollen, red and had begun to develop Peau d'Orange. I made an appointment with my family doctor the Friday after we returned, but there weren't any openings for 10 days. Sunday, I was looking on the Internet for "other causes of Peau d'Orange" and really began to appreciate how serious this was, as "Inflammatory Breast Cancer" became something that was no longer a distant text book memory, but a very likely diagnosis for me.

Diagnosis

On Monday, April 10, 2006, I called to make a more urgent appointment with my doctor, because there was obvious nipple retraction and skin retraction and I knew I couldn't wait. The nurse got me in to see my Family Doctor that afternoon. She had seen IBC before, so she knew right away what was going on and called the surgical oncologist (she had to leave a message) while I was still in the office. I saw him 2 days later, and he knew it was IBC as well. That day, I had a basic Mammogram which showed calcifications, a more detailed Mammogram to define the area, an Ultrasound, a chest X-Ray (which was normal) and several core biopsies of the area as well as some skin biopsies (I was "fitted in" on the radiologist's lunch break). The plan was outlined to me right from the beginning: chemo to contain the IBC, then radical mastectomy, then possibly more chemo and/or radiation.

Then, I waited until the biopsy results came in. I knew that they were going to be bad, but Jamie held on to the hope that "it" was just an infection or something relatively easy to treat; he hoped for it to be anything but IBC. I told the two people I worked most closely with that I suspected I had an advanced form of cancer and was awaiting test results, and began telling my psychotherapy patients that I "might be away for a while". One of my patients, a nurse, asked outright if it was "something serious" (her words) and began to cry when I stammered that I thought it might be.

As a professional courtesy of sorts, I guess to save me from having to wait for an appointment, the surgeon called me with the results, on Thursday afternoon April 20, 2006. I received the call between my last two psychotherapy patients of the day. Despite the fact that IBC was confirmed and that everything for me had now changed forever, I managed to see my last patient (for an hour). It took me at least twenty minutes to get the "now I have cancer... now I have cancer...now I have cancer" mantra far enough into the back of my mind to be able to concentrate on my patient. At the end of the session, I told her I would be away for a long time and that I would try to help her find another psychotherapist. I then changed my voice and e-mail return messages to reflect this, called Jamie, grabbed a few things and drove home, in a state I would call "suspended shock".

Even though I didn't know it at the time, because I thought I'd feel the urge to go back to work, I haven't worked since then. As soon as I got the phone call, I lost the "medical empathy" I needed to look after others. I began the "Physician, Heal thyself" path that I had always believed in. I had belonged to a group called "Physicians Health Action", which was focusing on helping ensure physicians were encouraged to find balance in their lives. I actually found it very difficult to accept "not working" without huge amounts of guilt, which still twinges now and then.

So, on with the story: Jamie was waiting in tears when I arrived home and kept saying "I thought we had all the time in the world....I want to be your husband and be by your side through whatever comes now". I called my friends, got one of my friends to cover for me teaching a craft class that night, called my parents and then Jamie and I cried, pretty much all night. Our worst fears had been realized, and we were reeling.

The next day, we woke up with resolve to face whatever we had to face, and my nickname "Debbie Warrior Princess" was coined. It took Jamie a few hours to shake off the feeling that I was "already gone", but he rallied relatively soon. This would actually become our pattern on hearing bad news: tears through an almost sleepless night, a brief sleep, Jamie looking at me like I was a ghost for half a day, and then we'd rally to fight again.

The morning of April 21, knowing we couldn't fight the battle alone, I sent out the following e-mail:

"Hello everyone,

I hate to do this by e-mail, but it's the quickest way to get the information out and I figured you all should know.

Yesterday, I got a confirmed diagnosis of breast cancer, left sided. It came up within the last three weeks and is an aggressive type, which requires chemotherapy before surgery and radiation.

We've been on a roller-coaster ride for the last little while but are now preparing for battle mode...so you can start calling me "Debbie, Warrior Princess" if you'd like. It will help me laugh and keep up the strength to fight! Jamie said to stop joking that we'll be making a film "My Left Tit", but I thought I'd get it in anyway!

I'll be at home for the next little while and am not sure if I'll be working during chemo, since I don't know how it will affect me. If you want to call, my home number is 457-0770.

I still plan on having the big brunch sometime as soon as possible, but there will be a much bigger focus on Pink than I had originally planned!!!

Take care,

Debbie"

I received so many supportive responses from that e-mail and from subsequent word-of-mouth that I was overwhelmed with a feeling that if support made a difference, I had a huge fighting chance. One of my great friends insisted on making 3 home-cooked meals for Jamie and me each week while I was on chemotherapy, AND she sent the word out to all of her card-making groups, who began sending beautiful and supportive hand-made and "regular" cards from all over the world (I've received well over 200 to date!) AND for our wedding, she made all of the invitations (but I'm getting ahead of myself!!).

April 22, Jamie took me out to dinner for what was to be our "Battle Feast" and proposed to me. Of course, I said yes, and we ate to excess and drank champagne to celebrate. We planned to pick out the "real ring" (Jamie had quickly picked out a "proposing" ring on Friday) on Monday.

The next morning, I had some belly pain, which I attributed to the excesses of the night before. When it didn't respond to antacids and OTC pain medications, and kept getting worse, I felt my belly and realized I could feel my liver edge. Jamie insisted on taking me to the emergency room, where we waited for six hours (a drawback of not doing what a normal patient may have done---call their doctor first—because I still wasn't used to being a patient. Had I called first, I probably wouldn't have had to wait so long.) Anyway, I saw another colleague (remember, I had gone to the local medical school and was still working in the university environment), who hadn't heard about my diagnosis (only a few people had at this point) but we both knew it had spread to my abdomen. Since it was very early Monday morning by now, he gave me a prescription for pain medication (I would only accept Tylenol #3, although he was willing to give me something much stronger) and booked an ultrasound for me later that morning and Jamie and I went home to sleep for a few hours.

We returned, and I had the ultrasound (I told them to do a "staging ultrasound" since one was booked for later that week). Another former colleague had to tell me that the cancer had already spread to my liver and spleen....and then I felt truly devastated. I later saw that the CT scan said that the liver lesions were "too numerous to count."

Despite that, I made Jamie take me to the custom jewelry shop so he could show me the engagement ring he wanted to order—I needed something positive to happen that day. The saleslady at the shop had heard some of the story when Jamie had gone in the previous Friday to pick out the "proposal ring" (apparently, he had walked in with determination and purpose, stating: "I'm looking to marry a gal"), and she was very warm and kind. Then we went home, cried, told our friends and family and followed what would become our "usual" pattern of response. My mother drove in to see me after I called her in tears and later told me that my father was a "basket case" when he heard the news. My parents and I had had some difficulties after my divorce in 2002 (bottom line: they had problems accepting that I was happy so soon after I left my ex-husband and didn't quite trust that I was wise in my feelings about Jamie) but we (my parents and I) reconciled in late 2004 (Thank God!!!!).

Treatment

Anyway, the appointment with our medical oncologist had already been arranged for April 26. As Jamie and I waited in the office to meet our medical oncologist…I should interrupt here to explain what will become the frequent use of "our" and "we": Jamie was true to his word and came to every appointment and test (other than regular blood work) that I had, right from the beginning. On one occasion, he had to leave an appointment that had run late, because he had a business meeting, but he was otherwise my "Warrior Prince"…anyway, we knew that the cancer had already spread and that things had changed, but the oncologist didn't know we knew. One look at his anguished face when he entered the room, and I quickly "reassured" him that we already knew the really bad news. I had been in similar positions before and needed to help him through it. He then explained that the overall treatment plan would shift from "curative" to "palliative," but that they would treat it very seriously, with strong chemotherapy (FEC 100= 5-FU (5-Fluorouracil), Epirubicin, Cyclophosphamide) and see how I responded. We hadn't received the hormone-receptor results yet, but he was encouraged that I might be estrogen-receptor positive, since some of my symptoms seemed to have settled after I had gone off the oral contraceptive pill (my only medication) at the beginning of April.

I started chemo on April 28 and would go on to have it every three weeks for a total of six sessions. Blood tests showed that my liver functions were severely reduced, so the Epirubicin dose was only 50 percent for the first three sessions. I was also given prophylactic medications to reduce side effects: Zofran (Ondansetron), Dexamethasone and Metoclopramide, which were given both intravenously just before the chemo, and as oral medications I took for up to three days after chemo. They worked well, although my oncologist later explained that he thought I had so few side effects because I was so sick with the cancer and metastases before starting chemo.

The FEC 100 seemed to work well, and after I stopped it in August of 2006, I went on Zoladex (Goserelin), a hormone treatment that put me into "medical menopause," which I give myself every 12 weeks. I began taking Aromasin (exemestane), an aromatase inhibitor that I take orally every day. I continue taking Pamidronate, a bisphosphonate, every three or four weeks to help reduce the risk of osteoporosis and also keep the bone metastases at bay.

My oncologist has measured my tumor markers, CA 15-3, since the beginning. They peaked at 1240 (normal is less than 30) after my first chemo session, and went as low as 70 in late December 2006, but then began to climb in January 2007. My left breast had also begun to swell again in early December, at first in an area in the upper part of my breast, which we thought might have been a cyst. An ultrasound showed that it was probably a lymph node. Then, the rest of the breast began to swell, and we feared the worst. However, CT and bone scans showed that the metastases were stable, suggesting that it was probably just local changes in the breast. After much discussion, I am booked for surgery March 1, with radiation to follow. Had there been any sign of progression of the metastases, I would have started with another bout of chemotherapy first.

As for the emotional aspects, and how we've dealt with all of this: The evening of my first chemo, a local church auxiliary's annual wine and cheese art show was being held. We had attended for the last three years and always picked up interesting art work, so I was hoping I'd feel well enough to go...luckily I did, and we came home with two paintings, fond memories of an evening spent with friends, and the sense that we could enjoy life despite the treatments. This "carpe diem (seize the day)" attitude has kept up our spirits and reflects a decision I made in 1999 and translated to my car's license plate in 2003 (as CRPDIEM).

Jamie is a videography producer and he began a series of "shoots" of me talking about my reaction to what was happening to me and also about my hopes for the future. I think we were both unsure how long I would live, and we wanted to get my thoughts and feelings on camera in case my son, who was living with his father in Ontario, needed to see them later. I think we did three or four of these "sessions," but we haven't been able to look at them…yet.

Although we were devastated and weren't sure how much time I would have, Jamie and I consciously decided that we would fight as hard as we could, work with the hand we were dealt, and live life to the fullest. We planned our wedding in July and worked fun around my chemo treatments…picnics out of town in the Mustang convertible he bought in the spring, day trips to the Annapolis Valley, and mini shopping sprees.

However, there were many anguished times when I blamed myself for "missing" the obvious signs that must have been there before they became so obvious—I am a physician, after all—I should have somehow known! I also felt guilty for not working, although my oncologist had said without hesitation that I shouldn't work and I had been prepared with private disability insurance, which would kick in by August. I used money from my retirement savings plans (RRSPs) to help get through the first few months without pay for many of our "extra" expenses. I would often say that my goal was to live long enough to use my RRSPs "legitimately"—at 65—and then I would start to cry, worried that I might not make it to 65.

It's a bit odd, though, that I never had any real "Why

me?" moments, even though I came close with my constant wondering about what caused this (was it my oral contraceptive, bad karma, a virus, my diet…basically, somehow or other, my fault?). I still wonder, in the hopes of finding a clue to improving treatments and finding a cure or finding ways to prevent IBC.

My diet hasn't changed much, since I've always had a hearty appetite and a fairly healthy diet as a true blue omnivore. I have tried to increase my intake of berries (which I have always enjoyed) and take multivitamins and grape extract when I can. I have reduced my beef intake somewhat but continue drinking red wine every now and then. I also try to walk daily and drink lots of water.

I also bought a whole bunch of books to help me through this: Bernie Siegel's *Love, Medicine and Miracles*; his *Faith, Hope and Healing*; *With The Help Of Our Friends From France: Stabilizing And Living With Advanced Breast Cancer* by Carol Silverander; *Advanced Breast Cancer: Holding Tight, Letting Go*, by Musa Mayer (which I haven't read yet); *Life in the Balance: My Journey with Breast Cancer* by Dr. Marla Shapiro (also haven't read yet!); *The Survivor Personality*, revised edition by Al Siebert (which I am currently reading and really enjoy).

My friends and family continue to support me as I fight this illness, I try to quote the mantra: "I do not fear you (the cancer); I am stronger than you" every day. I am working on ways that I can contribute locally to help others going through difficult times and hope that they will be meaningful.

Carpe Diem!

Ed. Note: Debbie Duerden McDonald, MD, died October 11, 2007. She was 42. She was instrumental in encouraging other IBC patients to tell their stories.

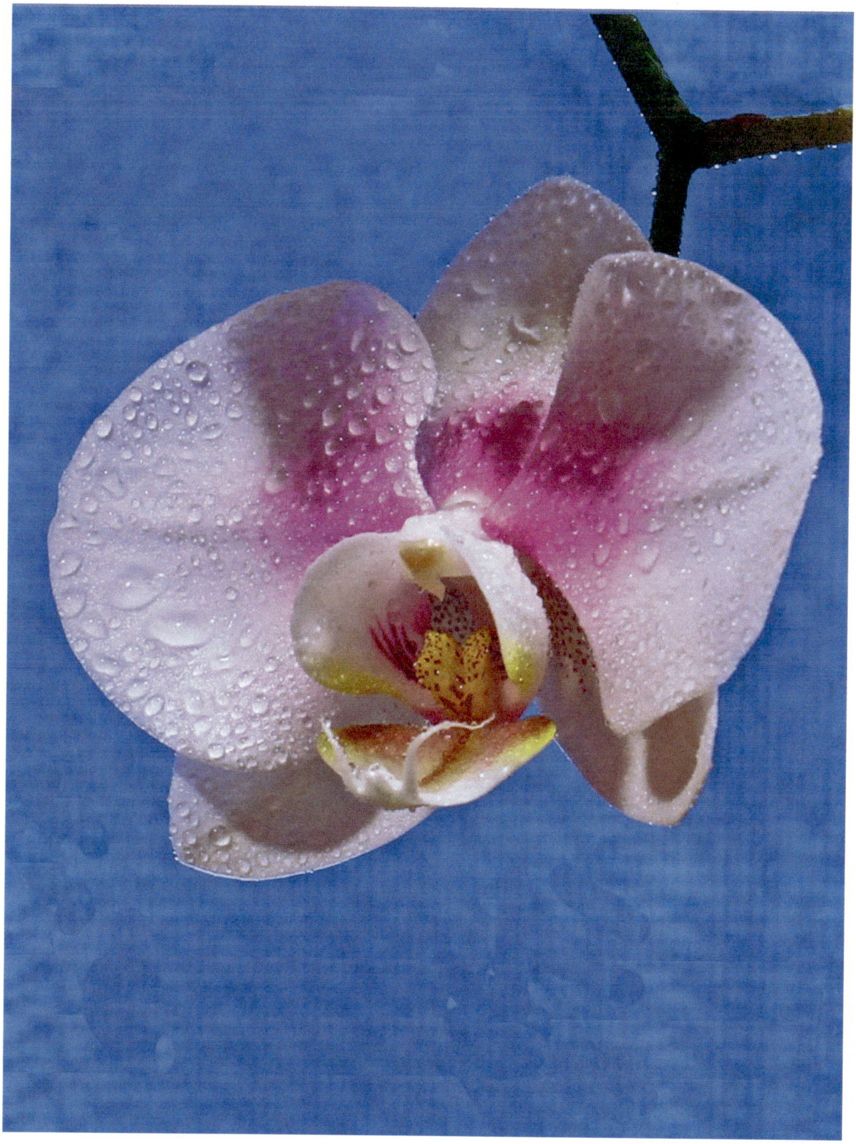

Tina's Story

There's a part of you that always remains a child, no matter how mature you get, how sophisticated or weary.
Barbra Streisand

The sunlight peeking through the curtains woke me. I wanted more sleep but the alarm clock was set to ring and I had a million things waiting for me at work. Tossing the covers off and giving my big beautiful Labrador "Black Bart" a pet and a hug, I headed for the shower. Always my shadow, Bart followed me into the bathroom and sat quietly while I turned the water on for my shower. Pulling my nightie over my head I felt a tugging sensation on my right breast. Instinctively I felt my breast and was shocked at how swollen it was. Looking in the mirror I was even more shocked to see how red and angry it looked. What had I done in my sleep? Had Bart stepped on me or banged his head into me and I didn't know it? Thinking back over the previous day of desk work and then a vigorous workout at the gym, I decided I must have pulled a muscle. That was it! I pulled a muscle and hurt one breast? Odd. How could that happen?

The shower felt good. The hot water streamed onto my sleepy face and spilled over my swollen breast. Out loud to the ever present Bart, I said, "I better be more careful, huh boy!" Wagging his tail in agreement, as he nosed the shower curtain back and watched me, his eyes glued to me, he gave a low bark to tell me all was good with the world.

It was April and the sunshine and rain were waking up all the flowers and the weeds, which would be attacked after work. The ever-present dust from the plowed fields around the house sat on the window sill that I dusted relentlessly, but never seemed to stay ahead of.

My bra was very tight as I dressed for work. Twinges of shooting pain from the swollen breast reminded me to keep an eye on what was happening. Reaching for the Tylenol with my right hand, the stabbing pain shot through my breast and took my breath away. Downing two pills should do the trick until the muscle calmed down.

Driving to work, I wished I was left-handed instead of right-handed as shifting the little Volkswagen was not an easy job that morning. But, after getting to work, the tall stack of loan documents to sort through quickly took my mind off anything else. The pain came and went all day, a constant reminder that something wasn't quite right, but by evening the pain seemed to ease. "Nothing to worry about," I said out loud to Bart as he laid his head in my lap later that evening.

June and July were hot in Eastern Washington and thanking the heavens for a home swimming pool, I jumped in every night after work. Mom and Dad had just bought a new boat and asked me to help christen her that July. My breast was still swollen, but thoughts of anything other than a pulled muscle taking longer than normal to heal I didn't tell Mom. She would just worry!

In August Mom mailed the pictures of the boat christening. As I flipped through them I stopped and stared at one with Mom and me sitting at the little dinette table on the boat. I had a tee shirt on and could see how swollen and lopsided I was. Mom hadn't noticed and I hadn't either, until visually I saw how much difference there was between the right and the left breast. It was later that evening that I took a good long look in the mirror and realized that my nipple had flattened and was starting to invert. Years of nursing training and I was being really stupid, waiting until now to decide I needed a doctor to check me out. Muscle problems didn't take this long to go away. Five months of absolute denial that this could be anything other than my original thought was really stupid. I got on the phone and made an appointment for the middle of September, which was the earliest I could get in. Maybe by then the swelling would be gone and I could cancel the appointment.

Diagnosis

On September 15th I walked into the office of my doctor and the nursing assistant came to take my vitals and ask what I was being seen for. I opened my shirt and showed her my still swollen breast and now totally inverted nipple. She put her pencil down and said, "I'll be right back." She didn't close the door completely and I heard her say to someone in the hall, "This patient is done"...my mind finished her sentence… "done for." I knew in my gut I was in trouble. I didn't have any lump, I had checked that repeatedly over the last six months.

"You need a mammogram," the assistant said, re-entering the room. Duh, I thought silently, as I put on the gown she had given me. Since it was the middle of the week, my mind was only half-heartedly on what was happening. Thinking of all the paperwork piling up at work, I just hoped this appointment would be quick. Wednesdays are hump day in more than one way when you are doing home loans for people. The end of the month was fast approaching and my mind was in gear for the work week, but not so much on a swollen breast. Infection, probably? Torn ligament, maybe, from lifting too many bar bells in the gym?

"Raise your arm and move closer to the machine," the mammography tech said. "Ouch…that hurts" I said as the plates pushed down hard on my very swollen appendage. "A man must have devised this torture machine," I said to the tech. "I'd like to meet the guy and stick *his* appendage in this machine." We both laughed and the female tech agreed.

Back in the room I sat and waited for the doctor and wondered why the mammogram had hurt so bad. Yeah, I was swollen, but the pain was excruciating when the plates mashed my body part. Being only 37 years old, I had never had this test, and hopefully wouldn't have to have it again for a very long time. Saying it was painful didn't even describe how bad the experience was. As I sat on the table in my gown, swinging my legs and thinking of work, a doctor came in that I had never seen before. She was tall and very elegant looking and dressed as though she had just walked out of a Chico's catalog. We exchanged pleasantries before she started asking me, "Why have you waited so long to have this checked out?" What could I say? "Stupid and way too busy," was my only true answer. She just shook her head and asked me to lie back on the table. Slowly she worked her fingers gently around my swollen and now very painful breast as she asked all the pertinent questions. I liked her immediately for her matter of fact way of getting down to the realities of my situation. "Your breast has all the clinical signs of Inflammatory Breast Cancer." "What in the world is that?" I asked, thinking it sounded more serious than I thought. "I don't have a lump so why would you think this could be cancer?" I said as I felt my stomach start to turn acid with the thought of what she was saying. "I'm only 37. How could I have breast cancer?"

A biopsy was ordered immediately, and before my appointment was over, I was sent to the surgeon's office where I had a punch, a fine needle aspiration, and a skin biopsy. I returned to the room where the oncologist would meet me. My breast was pounding with pain and I could hardly raise my arm after it was all over. "I will call you tomorrow and let you know the results," the doctor said, and with that...she left the room. The next day, Thursday, I was back in her office and hearing what no woman wants to hear. "You do have breast cancer, and this is the most aggressive of them all. I have ordered a PET scan and an MRI today, so I hope you have prepared to be here for quite a while." I hadn't of course, as this was not what I was prepared for. I needed to get back to work. By the end of the day, I was the last patient in the medical clinic. The doctor came in and sat down in front of me. "I am sorry to tell you this, but your cancer is Inflammatory Breast Cancer, and it has metastasized to your liver. This makes your stage of cancer stage four. We need to get you into immediate chemotherapy as fast as we can so we can hopefully slow this progression." She was talking fast now, and my mind was picking up only part of what she was saying. How many stages to cancer are there? What does stage four mean? Chemotherapy? Hold on, we are moving way too fast, I thought, but at the same time, even if I didn't know this doctor very well, I felt she really knew what she was doing.

Sitting in the parking lot of the clinic, the enormity of what I had just heard and been through engulfed me. I hated to cry, hated seeing others cry. But the tears came and I couldn't quit sobbing. My God, in just one small amount of time my world was upside down. Cancer. CANCER! But what in the world was Inflammatory Breast Cancer? All through nursing school and pharmacology training I had never heard of this. I wracked my brain for what seemed like forever as I composed myself for the long drive home. I prided myself on my memory and had had good grades all through my training. What had I missed? Where was it written you could have breast cancer with no lump? I couldn't doubt the biopsy, but was I so dumb not to realize after six months I could have something that could possibly kill me? Anger took the place of tears as I drove. "I'm not a statistic," I said aloud. The doctor's words floated in and out of my thoughts... "prognosis is not good with this type"..."mastectomy will follow months of chemotherapy"..."you will lose your hair from the chemo"...I looked in the rear view mirror and nervously laughed to myself. I hated my hair anyway, but then the tears started again. What the hell? Why me? I did everything to stay healthy, eating, exercise, everything. This is really happening, but why?

That night I called my mom. The hardest thing I had ever done was to tell her what had happened and what was going to happen. I prayed she didn't say what the surgeon and the oncologist had said: "Why in the world did you wait so long?" She didn't. "Can you come over please?" I asked. "I can't do anything. I am so sore from what they did today." "I'm on my way" was the only answer and three hours later we were standing at the gate holding each other with tears streaming. Standing in the hot sun with the dust of the farm swirling around us, I said, "Do you want to see it?" Not waiting for an answer, I opened my blouse and showed her my doubly swollen right breast with blood still oozing through the bandages where just hours before three separate biopsies had been taken. "I can't lift my arm or take a deep breath, it hurts so bad." She wrapped her arms around me, and in that moment I wanted her to take me home with her and make everything go away. For a brief moment, time seemed to stand still. Two human beings, five dogs, and a sea of emotion that somehow I knew the dogs could feel. They were still, standing quietly surrounding us. You don't ever see that. This was going to be a long fight, but I knew she was up for it, and I needed her to be strong. Tears weren't going to make this any better, so we agreed to keep them at a minimum, if possible.

Treatment

I laid out all the documents I had received from the oncologist. Places for her to sign so the doctor could talk to her (the wonderful HIPPA law, you know). The documents explaining that the drugs I would be taking were a trial:

Carboplatin, Taxol, and Herceptin. The side effects sounded brutal. I watched as Mom read each line, more than once asking if I was sure I didn't want a second opinion before beginning this journey, but I told her what I had decided. I looked her straight in the eye, looking for any sign I was making the right decision, or not. I had made up my mind and in a louder than normal voice, I said: "Mom, these drugs are either going to cure me or kill me. It's already in my liver, so...."

My mom was the computer person in the family, and she had immediately gone on the Internet to find out what this condition was. IBC, as it was called, had really bad statistics, especially at stage four. Mom had been a reporter for many years, and I literally begged her to start writing about this, as I was so shocked to find out that no one even knew what it was. "Mom, I am not a statistic...and this, uh, condition...is not going to define who I am. It isn't going to rule me."

"You do the research and just give me the highlights, but write and tell people because women need to know about IBC and how fast it can come on, and how young you can be to get it. Promise me...OK?" She promised.

The very next day I was sitting in a recliner in a private room starring wide-eyed at my mom. She didn't take her eyes off of mine because in my heart I knew she was waiting to see my reaction to what was going to begin. "I have kept my body away from drugs all my life and look at this. Look at all the poison." Bending down, she kissed my forehead and told me she loved me, and that she knew I was strong. As the first of the drugs began to trickle from the overhead bag, a tear escaped and slid down my face. "I hope I can be, but more, I hope you can be strong." I watched her jaw tighten as she said, "I will be little one, I will be."

"Good Lord," I said to no one in particular, but I was

staring into my mom's eyes when the first of the drugs started their march into my body. "I stayed away from drugs all these years, and now look at this," I repeated. "I'm getting a triple dose of this. I told you, this shit is either going to kill me or cure me, Mom, and I hope you are ready for whatever it brings." The nurse looked up at my mom, who was holding my free hand and stoically staring at her only daughter. I think the nurse thought my mom didn't have much emotion as she watched Mom sit straight up and just hold on. But I knew better. She had promised me no tears…and she was being my rod at that moment. I knew what was going on in her mind, at least I think I did…sorta along the lines of...this isn't real! She only said one thing to the nurse: "I'm sure glad we have good solid and strong Icelandic blood in our veins. We are going to need it."

Mom stayed with me for the first week, as the doctor said I needed someone to watch and keep tabs on my temperature after the first chemotherapy drugs were in my system. The first few days were fuzzy. I slept and drank tons of water and juice. Every time I even slightly opened my eyes, Mom had a huge glass of water with a straw and said, "Drink more." She was constantly sticking a thermometer in my mouth as the doctor had said to watch if my temperature went over 100.5. It never did. The extra drugs for the side effects made me very sleepy, so while I dozed off and on, Mom busied herself cleaning my house of the Eastern Washington dust that snuck into every crack it could. "Is my house dirty?" I asked her. "No sweetie…I'm just making work for myself, you rest." Which I did, for I don't know how many days. The physical and emotional drain on my system was the biggest shock. I thought I could tough it out, but the drugs to ward off the side effects were too much for me. Thankfully I didn't have really bad side effects, which I will attribute to the constant water being shoved down me by my overly vigilant mother. "I can't drink anymore, I will bust," I said more than once. "Yes you can, just go pee more often" was the repeated reply. "I know how much you hate to toss your cookies, so just keep washing out your system and maybe that won't happen." And it didn't. She was right. I called her Nurse Cratchet for over a week until I told her she could go home.

It took me a week to gather my mind and my body back to some semblance of normal, and work was the best medicine. The people at my job had become my second family and I didn't want to let them down. I also needed to keep working to remain insured. I wondered how people going through something like I was, uninsured, could possibly make it. All my work mates knew what I had been diagnosed with, but gladly they tried to keep their emotions in check, except my boss. She let her tears fall as she said, "whatever you need, we will work it out. If you need time off, just go. We will cover for you." And they did. A few weeks later they surprised me by bringing a single bed into a small office and set it up for me in case I needed to lie down. They were both business-like and tender. I felt like the luckiest person in the world to have these amazing people in my life. I had told them I didn't want any special treatment, and for the most part they went about the days as if everything were normal. But of course nothing was.

I had demanded that my infusions be on a Friday so that I had the weekends to recover. The doctor was very accommodating, so for eight long months we kept to a strict schedule. Monday mornings I would be at work and somehow my body (and my mind) were adjusting to the deluge of toxic chemicals being pushed through my body. Ironically there were times I looked forward to infusion Fridays. I had become close friends with my infusion nurse. She was so kind and caring—I felt very special. Since I wanted my life to not be ruled by the tag "cancer patient," she would talk about things totally remote to what was really happening. She was truly my savior on many occasions when my mind went into overdrive reacting to how my body was changing, how I hated my bald head, and how much weight I was gaining from the steroids. In the early months I would look in the mirror in the morning while I got ready for work and wonder if the person staring back at me would ever be normal again. I tried to make those thoughts fleeting, but it was hard. Because I was constantly seeing clients, I needed to look my best, and because I hated scarves, my hat collection became a coordination game with my wardrobe. It seemed I was constantly getting new clothes, as my weight was higher than I had ever seen it. Size 16 on my 5'4" frame was both embarrassing and uncomfortable. If it weren't for my family and work mates that kept my diminishing ego held up with comments like, "I love your hat" or "where do you find such nice clothes," I think I would have crawled into a hole and pulled the dirt right over me. My support system was just that...supportive and caring. But, after being the one who tried to "be there" for everyone, it was hard to accept that I was now the object that needed people to "be there" for me.

I had devised a little game with my clients. When a new client would come into my office and their eyes immediately shot to my hat, I would whip my hat off and show them my bald head. "I have breast cancer and I hate scarves." Getting that out of the way and leaving no room for more questions, I got on with my work. Watching people's eyes was like looking into their souls. They either looked sad or glad to get back to the paperwork in front of them. I learned very quickly that most people fear cancer, even when it doesn't affect them. Dealing with reality seemed less painful for everyone than their wondering why this woman was wearing a hat inside her office. Sometimes it was even comical to watch them wiggle around so they didn't have to stare at me.

Mom and I had long talks throughout the first months of treatment, and she suggested more than once, "Let's do something special, just you and me." We decided a Mexican Riviera cruise would be fantastic, so she booked the tickets and we were off on our adventure. I kiddingly said to her, "one bald chick and one old lady should be able to have a ball, don't you think?" And we did. There were some who thought we were nuts. My white blood count was lowered by the chemotherapy drugs, so some were worried that I would catch some bug on a ship. I didn't really care. Mom and I had been very real in our talks about "if the chemo didn't work." I felt there were things I wanted to do before I died…that I might die was a possible reality, just not one we talked about very often. A six-day cruise would take both of our minds off the reality of what was happening, and we both needed time…time for just mom and daughter. Time wasn't something either of us wanted to acknowledge, so for six glorious days we pampered ourselves and sailed away into the Pacific. We rode horses on the beach in Puerto Vallarta, shopped till Mom almost dropped in Cabo San Lucas, and swam with the dolphins in Mazatlan. I didn't have the energy that I was used to, but I could still out-walk Mom any day. Every morning on the ship we would sit on our little deck off our stateroom and just talk. I think we learned things about each other that we never knew. I guess you could call it a bonding time, but since we had had the luxury of being best friends for all of my adult life, had a cleaning business together, and started a mortgage business with the family, everything about the trip was like a pair of old souls just reveling in our alone time. Both of us joked about stowing away and not getting off the ship when it returned to Los Angeles…just sail away and never come back.

Eight months into treatment I received amazing news. They couldn't find any trace of Inflammatory Breast Cancer anywhere in my body. All the tumors in my breast, lymph nodes and liver had shrunk out of sight. I had beat this monster, it hadn't beat me. I was kept on the one drug that would keep the cancer from coming back, which was Herceptin. I still had to have this drug infused, but that was OK as long as I was now home free. As was the protocol with my type of aggressive breast cancer, I still had a single mastectomy which was followed with six weeks of radiation. The surgery, strangely enough, was a cake walk. I was in the hospital only overnight. Mom stayed with me for a couple of weeks to allow me to heal and help with the drainage tubes. That was a hassle but no pain. The radiation on the other hand was physically draining. I didn't stop work through the treatments, but the bed in the outer office called to me on more than one occasion. The exhaustion was debilitating, but I pushed through it with the help of my family and co-workers. I was on the home stretch and finally could see a big light at the end of this long journey.

For my birthday in December of 2005, Mom and I once again took off, but this time to Vegas to play and see Celine Dion on stage. It was a memorable birthday for me because two years prior I didn't think I would see forty. But there we were, walking the streets of Las Vegas, shopping, eating fantastic food, and of course gambling a bit, and then there was the amazing night we watched and sang along with our favorite singer. Life was good. My hair had grown back and I was feeling so good I could hardly believe what my body had been through.

In February of 2006 I began to feel an intense pain in my shoulder blade. I was staying with Mom when I first felt it. "Can you rub my shoulder?" I asked her one night. "I feel like I pulled a muscle." Unfortunately no amount of massaging helped the pain, so at my next appointment with my oncologist I mentioned the shoulder blade. I was whisked off to a CT Scan, and was immediately demoralized to find out my liver tumors were showing up again. “We are going to add something to the Herceptin infusion,” my oncologist said. “Great, I just got my hair back and here we go again.”

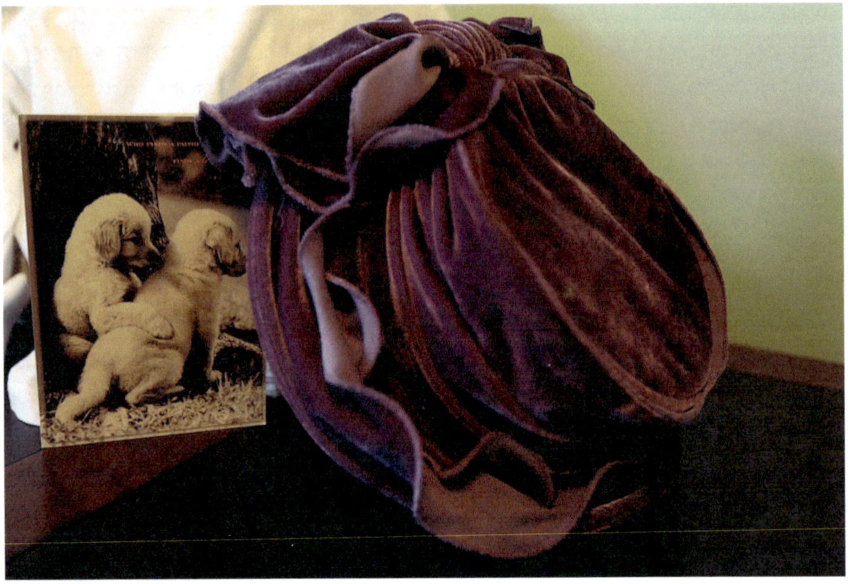

The hat that Tina wore, shown with a photo of Labrador puppies, which she loved

Tina’s Mom’s Story

“Mom I need to tell you something,” my little girl said into the phone. “Oh man, am I in trouble?” I said jokingly.

“Mom, I have cancer.”

My free hand shot to my chest as I said, “You what?”...“I have breast cancer”... she hesitated then said, “I have the kind that I’m gonna die.” I couldn’t speak. I could hear the blood pounding in my ears and she said, “Mom, are you there, are you OK?”

“Me?” I said half bent over feeling like I wanted to throw up. “I should be asking you that.” I honestly couldn’t think of one thing to say. I was numb. After a long silence, closing my eyes, I said, “When did you find this out?”

“Just today,” she said, then a rush of words…“I’ve known something was wrong for quite a while but couldn’t find a doctor…they say it is Inflammatory Breast Cancer, and it’s already in my liver…have you ever heard of it?” Still clutching my throat, I said almost vacantly, “No.” Another long silence. I felt blank…I couldn’t talk…there were no tears...just a deep hollow feeling in the pit of my stomach. “Mom, are OK?” she said again. “Can I call you back,” were the only words I could muster at that moment. “I’ll be here,” she said in a low, almost monotone voice.

As I hung up the phone, my husband said, “What was that all about? You are white as a sheet.” “Tina just told me she has breast cancer. I’ve never heard of what she said.” I felt like I was floating. I went to the back room and switched on the computer, and staring at the blank screen, I could feel my heart racing. I typed in “Inflammatory Breast Cancer” and what I read finally pushed the held-back emotions and tears to the surface. I cried like a baby. Brian, my husband, walked in, looked at the screen, and put his hand on my shoulder. “Are you sure this is what she said she had?” I stood up and went into his arms and the crying slowly subsided. He said nothing, just held me.

“I need to call her back” I said, “but I don’t want to be crying, she hates that.” I called her back and she picked up on the first ring. “Mom, are YOU OK!” she said in a much louder, stronger voice. “I’m as good as can be expected. I just looked up what you told me.”

“It’s bad, Mom, really bad. I’ve never heard of it either. Not in nursing school, nowhere. They took three biopsies and I am so sore I can hardly lift my arms. I hate to ask you, but can you come over?" There was no hesitation now as the shock was waning. "I'll toss some stuff together and be right over," I said trying very hard not to cry. "No, Mom, I need to get some sleep, come in the morning, please. Maybe you should have Brian drive you," she said. "No, I'll be OK...I will see you first thing in the morning. I love you kidlet." "I love you too," she said quietly.

The long drive over the mountains gave me time to think. Breast cancer. She was only thirty-seven years old. This had to be a mistake. Thinking back over what I had read on the computer earlier, the statistics for surviving this type of breast cancer were not good. And because it has metastasized, she was stage four, which was the worst case scenario. How could this be? She was so healthy and active, always taking care of herself, much better than I. The thoughts were a jumble...how was I going to handle this? How was I going to react? Tina hated to see me cry, which I knew only too well, so I needed to fight the emotions and be strong. How I was going to do that, I had no clue. The harder I thought, the harder I pushed on the gas pedal, backing off when I realized I was going over 80. Getting in an accident right now would really be stupid. I needed to be in one piece for her. My little girl...my baby...the tears blinded my vision as I slowed the car and again tried to compose myself.

As I drove up the gravel drive to my little girl's home, my stomach and mind were churning, both with anxiety and fear of what lay ahead. I turned the car towards the big cattle gate and saw her standing there, and could tell immediately she was in intense pain. Her five Labradors' sat quietly by her side as she motioned for me to get out of the car. Normally, she would have opened the gate, but not today. She couldn't. My own heart was pounding so hard I could hear it in my ears....I wanted to bawl, to run to her, to cry, but knew I couldn't. I had to be strong. Oh Lord, I will never forget that moment as long as I live.

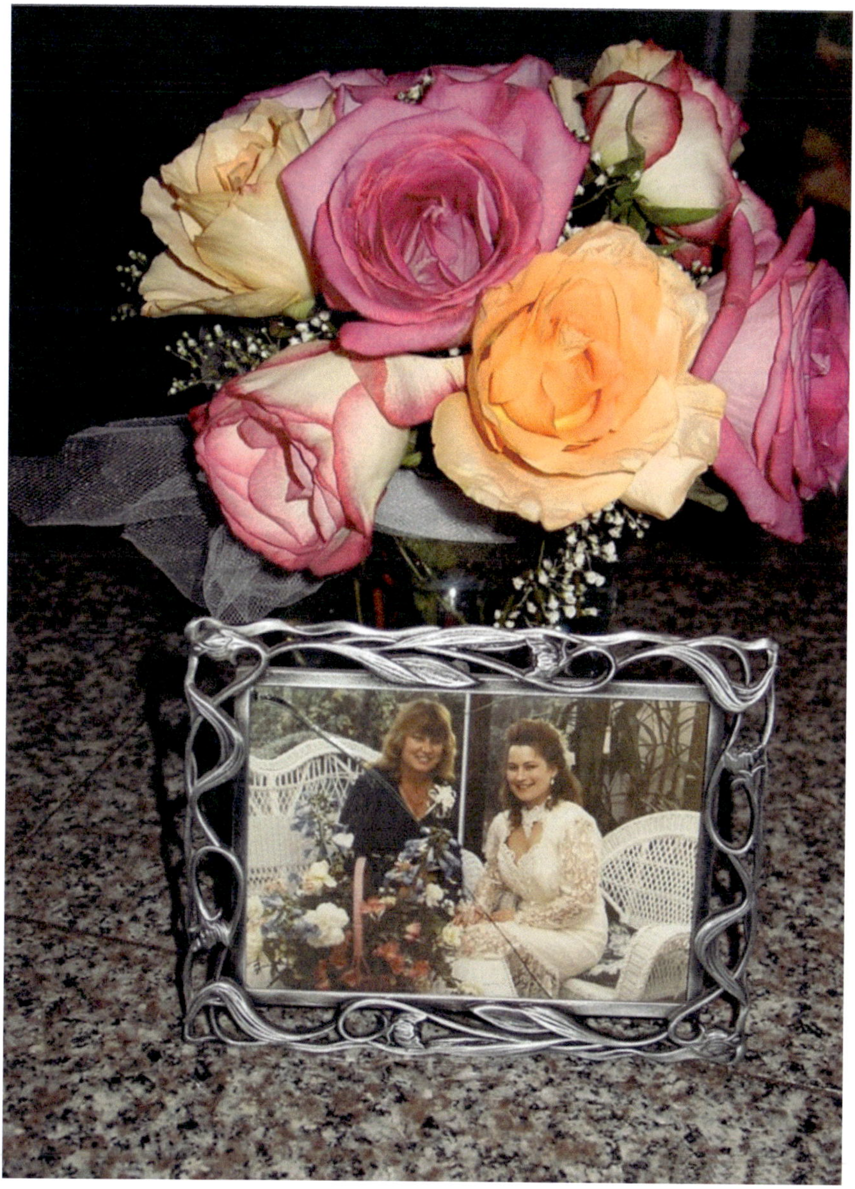

The very next day she was sitting in a recliner in a private room starring wide-eyed at me. She didn't take her eyes off of mine, because in my heart I knew she was waiting to see my reaction to what was going to begin. "I have kept my body away from drugs all my life and look at this. Look at all the poison." Bending down, I kissed her forehead and told her I loved her, and that she was strong. As the first of the drugs began to trickle from the overhead bag, one shiny tear slid down her face...."I hope I can be, but more, I hope you can be strong." My inner voice was screaming, "Why not me, God, why my little girl? Please! I know I am being selfish, but please don't take her from me."

Ed. Note: Tina passed away on August 29, 2007.

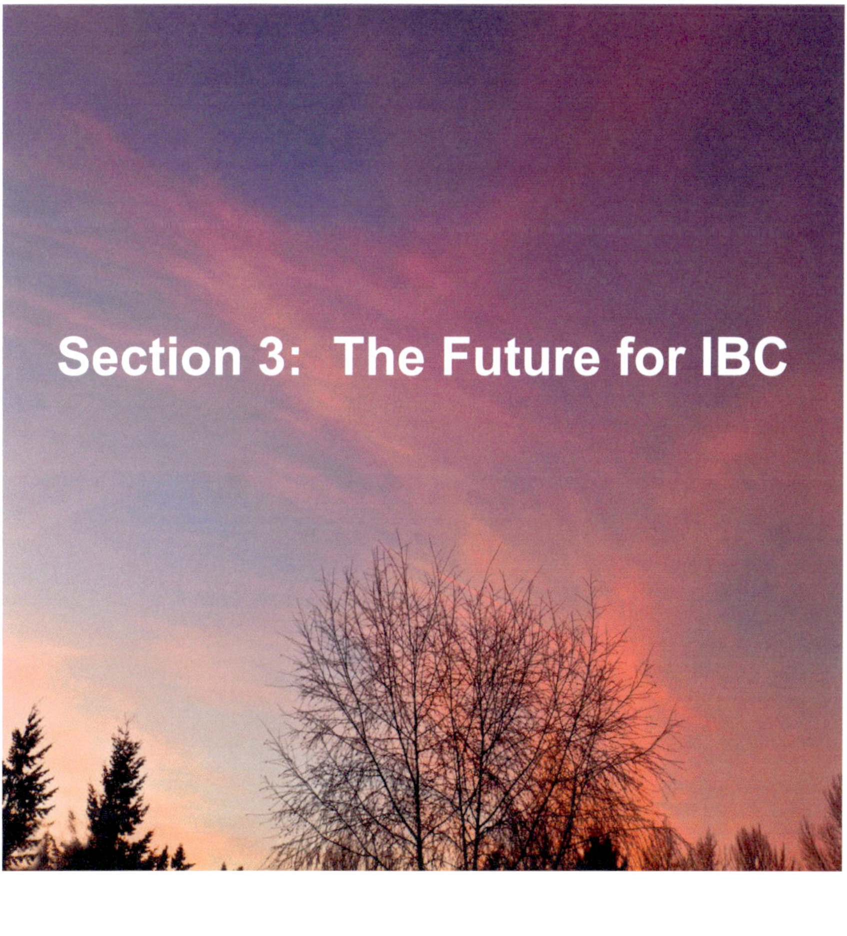
Section 3: The Future for IBC

A Dream, A Mission

By Dr. Massimo Cristofanilli

A man may die, nations may rise and fall, but an idea lives on.
John F. Kennedy

It was a cloudy morning in Houston. I woke up, looked outside the window, and realized it was going to be another warm and humid day. I got my kids ready as usual and I drove them to school. For some reason I felt sad and had a sense of anxiety that I could not explain. It seemed like I was on autopilot and the outside world was passing me by without giving me emotions or catching my attention. I needed to be in the hospital quickly because I had a clinic to start. I had been focusing recently on an aggressive form of breast cancer called inflammatory breast cancer (IBC) and most of my patients have been diagnosed with this devastating disease. Sometimes I get depressed because I really do not know what to do besides using the most effective and aggressive treatments.

My chairman has given me the responsibility of designing a new clinical study for IBC and I think I can use this opportunity to prepare something really new, but, where do I start? Our cancer center, even if large, has taken four years to enroll 43 patients in a clinical trial! This is far too slow for me. Moreover, for some reason, I believe I need to find a way to learn more about the disease and—dealing with such a rare condition—I think the most effective approach would be to have the opportunity to bring more IBC patients here. This is a simple and interesting idea, but how can it be realized?

I arrived at the office and turned on the computer to

look at the list of patients for today's clinic. I have two new patients in the morning and 12 follow-ups. I wondered if either of the new patients is actually an IBC case. I looked at the names and ages: Morgan Welch, 24 years old, from Florida. She is really young and is coming from out of town. She must have a serious problem. I put on my coat and closed the door behind me. I had a heavy feeling while walking down the long walkway. I had one more chance to look outside before entering the clinic. The clouds were dark gray and made me think it would be another oppressive and difficult day, but, strangely, I started to feel an inner peace. Entering the clinic felt like crossing an invisible line and going toward my destiny, and I felt a strange sense of happiness. Interestingly, I had had such feeling one other time in the past and I later realized that the episode had changed my life.

I had been a young physician who had just completed medical school and had started my training in oncology in my home country, Italy. I had taken that specialty very seriously because my father died of cancer and I wanted to have the chance to learn about it and find better ways to treat it. I had started in a university hospital in the medical oncology department under the direction of a talented mentor, particularly for breast cancer, Prof. Alberto Pellegrini. He really believed in me and appreciated my interest in research, and so he gave me the chance to work closely with him in private practice. During that time I was focused on my training and new responsibilities, but I also found time to fall in love with a younger colleague and get married. We came back from our wonderful honeymoon and we were ready to start working again as usual.

On our first day back,the moment that we stepped into the office at the day-hospital, I felt extremely uneasy and almost wanted to run away. What has happened? I have been here for two years and I have learned everything that I know in this place. Everyone has been supportive and we have friends that were with us celebrating just three weeks ago at our wedding! I had to focus for a moment and try to continue as if nothing were happening because I did not want my wife to see that I was uneasy. Eventually, I was able to start working again and finish my clinic. At home, I wanted to spend time with my wife and did not want to talk about this episode. Maybe it is just something momentary in my head and it will be gone in the morning. The following day, I wanted to go in earlier and arrive before anyone else to find out if I was back in my normal state of mind. I entered my office and ran to my desk to sit down. I looked around and everything seemed strange and almost unrecognizable.

What is going on? How can I continue like this? I decided to go to our meeting room to have the chance to chat with some of my friends, but they have not arrived yet. I sat down and looked around for something to do and my attention was drawn to a scientific journal, *Seminars in Oncology*. I started reading the first few pages and it was extremely interesting. I spent the next hour reading. I was so engrossed that I could not think about anything else. I read all the articles and then went back to the authors list. They were all from centers in the US. That's it! I needed to find a way to move to the US to be able to do what I really liked doing, clinical research! From that moment on, I was focused on doing everything it would take to realize my dream, and on June 4, 1993, approximately four years from that day, I departed from Rome to start my new adventure. My wife and I said goodbye to our families and our secure life to go toward the unknown, but I felt this was the right thing to do, no matter what would happen. And now, while I was entering the clinic, a question was coming to me: I had the energy to come to this great center and realize my dream, but what is my mission? Have I found it yet?

I sat down to read Mrs. Welch's story and it was really sad. She had just gotten married approximately six weeks ago, and in the last ten days her life completely changed. She found diffuse redness and skin edema in her right breast that was quite suspicious of IBC and she was concerned about it. Furthermore, she had complained of diffuse bone pain, particularly concerning in her thoracic spine. This was quite a terrible situation. I wondered if I could find something effective for her. Would I be able to go into the room and find some inspirational words to relieve her fears?

I have no time to think about this anymore. My nurse asked me, "What are you going to do with her? What kind of treatment?" She has been my assistant for several years and by now almost knows my answer. "You know I never decide about any treatment before seeing my patients. I need to look at her eyes and feel what is going to be right for her." I walked toward the exam room with a heavy heart. I knocked on the door and opened it. In front of me was a young couple holding hands. Morgan's mom was also in the room. I introduced myself and started to ask questions. Morgan appeared extremely frightened and was almost in tears. She first wanted to know if she had IBC because doctors had not been very clear about the diagnosis and then, of course, she wanted to discuss treatment and prognosis. I do not remember much. I was able to lie to her, and I saw Morgan becoming more relaxed. She trusted me and she would have done everything I would have suggested to her.

We treated her very aggressively and she appeared to respond quickly. We were able to bring her to surgery, complete radiation treatment, and start tamoxifen. We hoped that her disease would remain under control for some time, but it did not. The disease continued to progress into the nodes and pleura and she started to have more bone pain. We tried a few more treatments with mixed results, and then she had brain metastases. It was becoming more difficult at each visit to provide her with some relief and hope. The disease was taking control and we had no means to stop it. She was finally admitted to the hospital for comfort care. I visited her one last time. Her face was disfigured by the steroids and she could barely talk and breathe, but she was able to whisper a few words that would change my life: "Thanks for all you have done. I want you to promise me that you will continue to fight this terrible disease so that other women do not have to suffer." I looked at her for the last time and I said firmly, "I promise you. I will do everything I can." I hugged her and then waved goodbyc one more time while closing the door. I was extremely sad in a way that I have rarely been. I started writing my final note on her chart, and then, I understood. I had a mission now. I needed to find a better way to fight this terrible disease. My heart felt lighter and I was walking fast toward the office. I knew I could do this and the path was now very clear to me.

In the following months I worked extremely hard. I do not know exactly how I was able to pull off organizing this new project, that of creating a specialized IBC clinic. I must have had a superior force watching after me. First, I assembled a team of colleagues and explained to them what I felt was necessary to do. I remember sitting in a meeting room trying to convince them that I will find the resources and start doing research on IBC. They were supportive but skeptical at first, considering their past experience and the lack of institutional support. Next, we needed to open a specialized clinic that would try to understand the peculiarity of IBC by increasing the possibility of clinical observations and samples collection. I got in touch with Patti Bradfield, a tough and determined woman whose daughter was fighting this disease. She was looking for a chance to increase education and awareness of IBC. It seemed the perfect match. Many women helped in making this clinic possible and I will always be grateful to

Patti and Timothy Jennings, Pam Jones, Fredika Robertson, and the entire team of IBC ambassadors and researchers. I remember the idea of a specialized clinic was not initially accepted by my colleagues in the department and by the institution, and I had to fight to have this project realized. Nobody would believe that the largest breast cancer department in the US needed a specialized IBC clinic to focus on this aggressive disease.

On October 26, 2006, we inaugurated the IBC clinic with women and patients from all over the world. Subsequently, we dedicated the clinic and research program to Morgan as a symbol of a young and courageous IBC victim. Moreover, we were able to organize the International Conference on IBC that brought together clinicians, advocates, and researchers devoted to the disease. Approximately 200 participants from various continents attended this first event. I was proud to see the growing attention to—and the research interest in—this disease. I could now move to another institution to take my mission to the next level.

Patti and I are in constant contact with the goal of helping women everywhere. Our understanding of IBC has increased significantly and I believe we are getting closer to finding the cause and have more potentially effective treatments. Unfortunately, many physicians are still not properly educated, and women continue to be neglected or misdiagnosed. We need to speak with a stronger voice, but at least we are now focused on our specific priorities. I now know what my mission is, and I will not give up till I have kept my promise to cure this disease.

—Dr. Massimo Cristofanilli

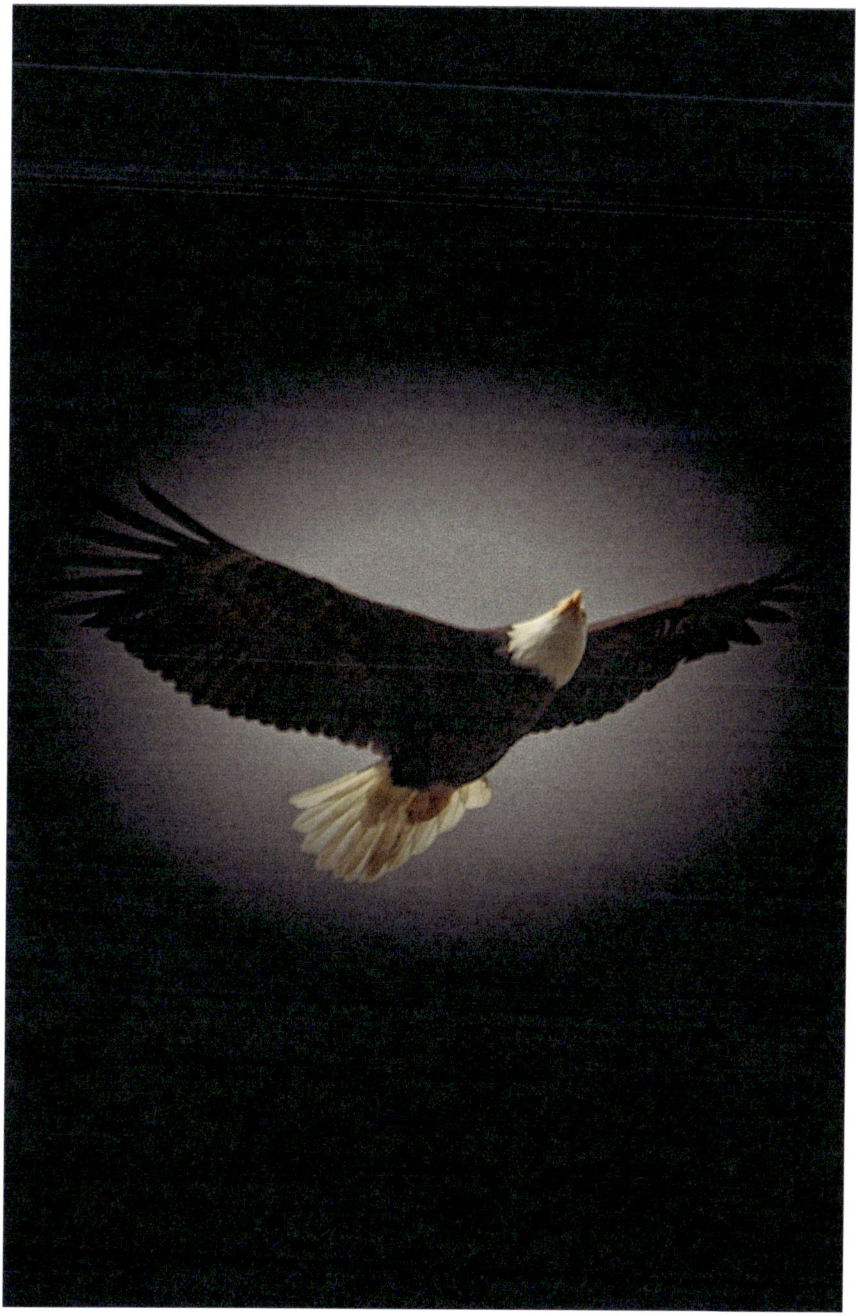

What We've Learned

The women who have had IBC have given us valuable information about diagnosis, treatment, and overall feelings of well-being. Here are some of the things we've learned from their stories:

Diagnosis

We are told to look for a lump and to get mammograms. We are not told there can be an undetectable mass that indicates inflammatory breast cancer.

ANY DIFFERENCE in your breast, AT ANY AGE should be looked at by a doctor who knows about IBC. There are still many doctors and other health professionals who have not heard of IBC because it used to be rare. However, the incidence of IBC is rising at an alarming rate.

Diagnostic Tests

Karen's oncologist commented that just because a PET scan shows clear doesn't mean the body is clear...that it takes billions of cancer cells to show a small area on the scan.

Medical Advice

Marijanne requested a double mastectomy but was told there was a less than 5% chance cancer would go to the other breast. However, she did develop IBC in her other breast. You are the patient and it is your body. It is up to you to decide what risks you want to take.

Bedside Manner

Joan's primary physician told her to see a surgeon, but did

not explain why. Doctors do not always communicate well. It is up to you as the patient to ask questions and demand answers. Don't let the medical establishment keep you in the dark.

Nutrition

Joan's daughter, a believer in home remedies using herbs and supplements, had purchased the book *Beating Cancer with Nutrition* by Patrick Quillin. Using this book as a guide, she made a list of supplements which Joan started taking several times a day when she started the chemotherapy. Joan believes that doing so helped improve her energy level and state of general health.

Radiation Burns

Joan found that 2nd Skin Moist Burn Pads applied to radiation burns were a life saver. She used these for several weeks while the area healed.

Spiritual and Psychological Support

Sandy found that the books of Bernie Siegel, MD, were uplifting. Dr. Siegel, a surgeon, writes about tapping the body's inner wisdom and capacity for self-healing. His success with patients is often called "miraculous." Dr. Debbie Duerden McDonald also listed books she thought would help.

Insurance Issues

Rich and Doracina had to search for a medical facility that was compatible with their insurance coverage. Make sure that your insurance covers the cost of treatment.

Goodbye Is Not Forever

By Patti Bradfield (Tina's Mom)

The room was dark, curtains closed to shut out the blazing Eastern Washington sun. My baby girl lay still in the bed with her faithful Lab close beside her. I took a stick with a pink sponge, dipped it in the water glass, and passed it gently across her parched lips. She opened her eyes and said, "Can we go to the beach?" Chocking back a cry I knelt down next to the bed and ran my hand over her cool forehead. "Sure we can," I lied. "The weather is beautiful for a stroll on the beach."

She was rail thin from the inability to eat, but her belly looked like she was nine months pregnant, with her liver so swollen it was pushing on her stomach and making it impossible to keep any nourishment down. Morphine was the only saving grace for the pain she felt and sleep seemed almost a savior for her.

It was August and the heat was unbearable during the day but the nights were wonderful. I would wheel her out to the patio in the evening and we sat for hours one night just looking at the stars and talked about better times, when she was young. Her baseball games, the horses we had, funny memories of picking blackberries together until our lips were purple and our buckets only half full.

It was a Saturday night, I remember. The stars looked as if you could reach up and touch them. Mother and daughter sat looking up to the heavens, trying to name off the constellations. "Are you going to be OK, Mom?" My mind snapped back as if out of a dream. "OK about what?" I asked. "When I'm gone?" My heart was pounding and I wanted to scream...but I didn't. I lied. "And where are you going?" She just smiled at me, but we both knew what was so close to happening that it couldn't be said aloud. I reached out and took her hands and said, "I love you kidlet, with all my heart and soul." "I know Mom, I love you too."

Wednesday morning, just four days later, at 3:05 am, my beautiful little girl went to sleep. Quietly, peacefully, the same way she had led her life. In dignity and grace, waiting until we all left the room. She had removed the oxygen tube from her nose, crossed her hands on her chest, and just went to sleep. My last memory was of a half smile of peaceful sleep as I kissed her one last time and let the pent up tears fall like a roaring waterfall. Again I asked God why my child and not me. What did he want from me?

A week passed. The memorial to her precious life was put together with so much love by her wonderful work mates, that I know she was proud. Her dear friend Ryan had put together a CD of pictures of her life, which was so fitting and wonderful. Everyone told me how she had always put others first, never herself.

And that was true.

Another week passed and I went alone, one more time over the mountains to gather her things and take home so much of what her life had been: mementos, pictures and albums, clothes. As I drove back towards the mountains that day, my van laden down with her belongings, I decided to sing along with a Barbra Streisand song that my little girl and I had always sung together. The tears stopped and my singing was loud along with the tape that was blaring. I could hear nothing but the song and my own voice…when suddenly I heard another voice. "I have her, Patti, she is with me and she is OK."

I slammed on the brakes and pulled to the side of the road turning off the music. I sat very still and waited to hear what I had heard just moments before. I knew the voice. It was my baby's grandmother, gone just five years before. I sat in silence and strained to hear her voice again, but it was gone. I don't know how long I sat there, but deep inside I felt a calmness, a warmth, and yes, I guess, a finality. She was OK. We would all be together again one shining day.

— Patti Bradfield, 2007

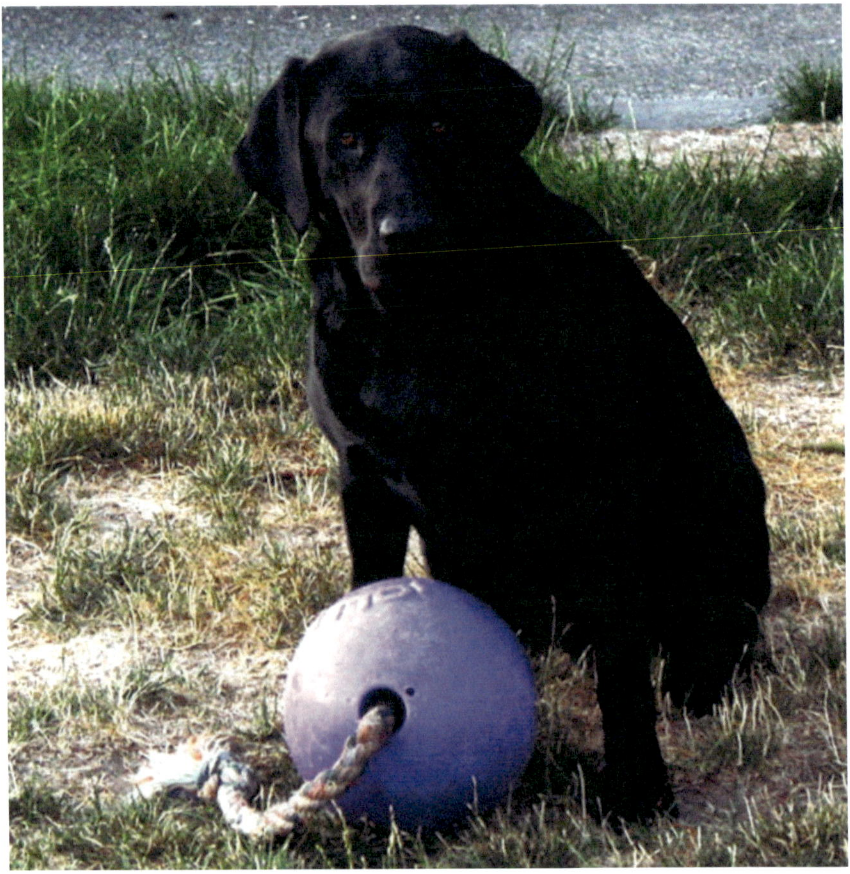

Tina's dog BooBoo waits to play with her.

Epilogue

Dr. Cristofanilli went forward and in 2006 opened the first-of-its-kind Inflammatory Breast Cancer Clinic inside the Nellie B. Connelly Breast Center at the MD Anderson Cancer Center in Houston, Texas. In 2010 he opened a second IBC clinic at Fox Chase Cancer Center in Philadelphia. He continues to research IBC and treat patients, with an insatiable need to find the cause and cure for this devastating disease. Because of more effective treatment, and particularly with the use of anti-estrogens and Herceptin, the percentage of women living free of disease for more than 10 years continues to increase.

Patti Bradfield, Dr. Cristofanilli, and Jenee Bobbora started the Inflammatory Breast Cancer Foundation (www.eraseibc.com) in May of 2007 to educate the public and the medical community about this misunderstood, misdiagnosed, and under funded research of IBC. They all continue to this day with volunteers of lay people and physicians who want to see an end to this...the untold story, that needs to go to the front of the line. For it is believed if this monster of a disease can be cured, other less aggressive breast cancers will also be just a memory.

That is our hope. That is our goal.

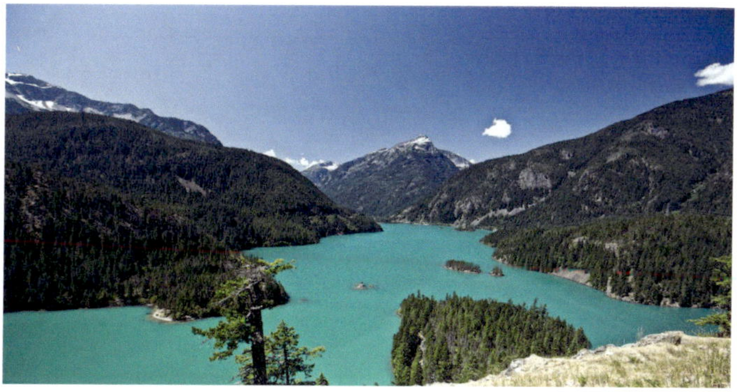

The IBC Foundation

The Inflammatory Breast Cancer Foundation (www.eraseibc.com) is a group of concerned citizens who came together with the hope of making a difference in the way Inflammatory Breast Cancer (IBC) is perceived by both the general public and the medical community.

Our ranks come from IBC patients, physicians, the media and those affected by IBC. Advocates and patients came from such places as Idaho, Washington State, Illinois, and London, England, in 2006 at the opening of the first IBC clinic in Houston, Texas. The advocates and doctors had a vision that culminated in the first-of-its-kind facility at MD Anderson Cancer Center.

Our mission is to change the perceived notion that all breast cancers have a lump. The medical community has not been educated to a degree where they can catch this deadly form of breast cancer earlier than stage IIIB. This is not acceptable.

We will do a national canvas of medical continuing education seminars, radio shows, television, and in-person interviews and reach as many people as possible to spread the word that there is more than one type of breast cancer, and that IBC can be deadly if not diagnosed properly. Countless women are fighting their own health care physicians to get a proper diagnosis, which has to stop. Through education and awareness, this can change.

Among our supporters are men and women who have lost wives, sisters, mothers, and daughters. We all know that regular breast cancer has been researched and many good things have come from what other grass roots organization's have done. We all know what the Pink Ribbon stands for, that women and men should look for a lump.

Now we need to educate with every medium that is earthly possible that there is a breast cancer that we have not been told about.

And we will.

"Women with IBC are warriors, not patients or survivors....Their passion to stop IBC has directly saved the lives of countless women by raising awareness. Because of them, the number of researchers studying this disease continues to increase and the scientific community is becoming more aware of the urgency underlying this aggressive cancer. Women with IBC often feel isolated and disenfranchised from the rest of the breast cancer community....IBC has a 5-year disease-free survival rate that is less than half of that for non-IBC. Thus any improvement would be welcomed by the IBC community."

— Dr. Kenneth Van Golen

About the Authors

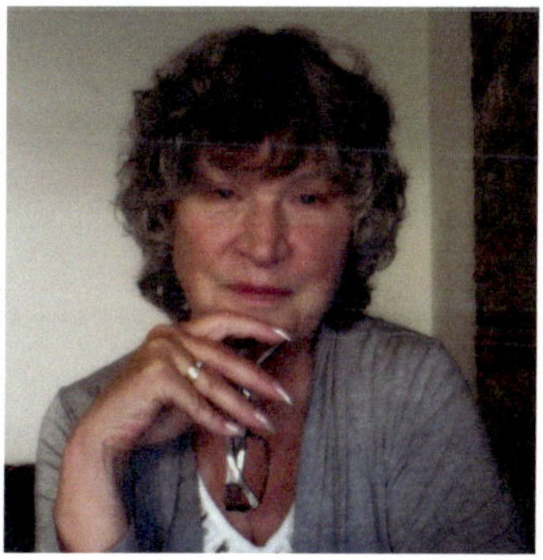

Patti Bradfield started her writing and photographic career 35 years before her daughter was diagnosed with IBC. As an investigative reporter, she pushed into every corner of news and publications to educate everyone about this disease, which is killing women at an alarming rate. Patti has been working with IBC patients since 2003, when her journey began with her daughter, helping them find doctors that would not only listen to their pleas, but actually be knowledgeable about IBC and how to treat it properly. Together with Dr. Cristofanilli and Jenee Bobbora, Patti founded The Inflammatory Breast Cancer Foundation. She also started an Internet radio show, *IBC Facts & Fallacies*, with the foundation's secretary, Peggy Stephens. The show is now into its sixth year. Patti has retired from the foundation but remains a strong advocate for women who need help, as well as a loud voice in the medical community where, in some places in the United States, IBC is still neither diagnosed nor treated properly.

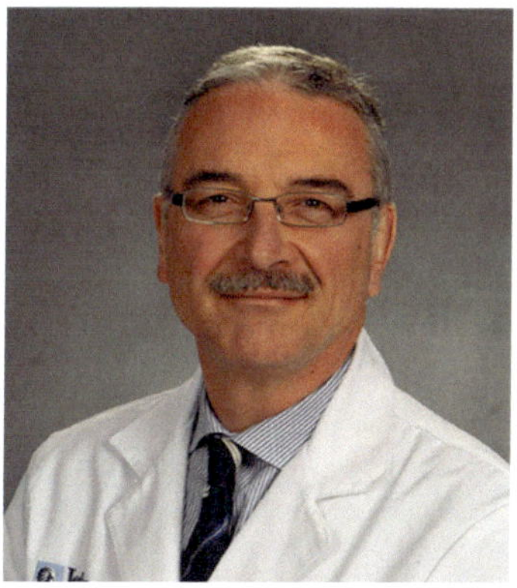

Dr. Massimo Cristofanilli graduated from the University "La Sapienza" in Rome and completed medical oncology training in Italy. He came to the United States with the intent of pursuing his dream of focusing on patient-centered clinical and translational research in breast cancer. He completed an internship and residency at Cabrini Medical Center in New York. He then completed a fellowship at the University of Texas MD Anderson Cancer Center. Dr. Cristofanilli's concept of team science and multidisciplinary research and care have been applied to IBC since 2006, when he founded the world's first IBC clinic: the Morgan Welch Inflammatory Breast Cancer Program and Clinic at MD Anderson. The clinic was dedicated to a young woman who had lost her battle with IBC. He continued to apply those principles when he moved to Philadelphia, first at the Fox Chase Cancer Center and now at Thomas Jefferson University, where he is currently the Director of the Breast Care Center. Dr. C., as most IBC patients call him, is married and the father of two children. His passion is to find the root cause of IBC and make sure women get the best of care that science can give them.

Made in the USA
Columbia, SC
30 December 2024

50889989R00073